# The Double Pandemic: COVID-19 and Misinformation in the Digital Age

Sharlin

First Printing, 2024

## Table of Contents

Page


1 Introduction ... 1
2 Relevance and Background ... 4
3 Framing Theory ... 15
3.1 Origins ... 18
3.2 The Power of a Communicating Text ... 21
3.3 Function of Frames ... 24
3.4 Emphasis vs. Equivalence Framing ... 28
3.5 Framing Effect ... 30
3.6 When the Power of a Communicating Text Meets the Power of the Oval Office ... 31
3.6.1 Cascading Network Activation ... 33
3.6.2 All Thought is Physical ... 34
3.7 When the Power of a Communicating Text Meets the Power of Digital Media ... 37
3.7.1 The Hybrid Media System ... 37
3.7.2 Are New Media Logics Redefying Power? ... 40
3.7.3 From Twitter to Traditional Media ... 45
4 Literature Review ... 49
4.1 Trump's Communication Style ... 49
4.1.1 Populism ... 49
4.1.2 A Man in the Street Communication Style ... 51
4.1.3 Direct Causation ... 53
4.1.4 Political Incorrectness ... 54

4.1.5 Hyperbole ... 55
4.1.6 Insult Politics and Mocking Rhetoric ... 56
4.2 Framing The COVID-19 Pandemic ... 58
5 Methodology ... 71
5.1 Context and Time Period ... 71
5.2 Sampling ... 74
5.3 Twitter Elements ... 76
5.4 Data ... 79
5.5 Typology ... 79
6 Results ... 85
6.1 Epidemic (January 24 – March 10, 2020) ... 85
6.2 Pandemic (March 11 – September 28, 2020) ... 88
6.3 Pre-election Period (29, September - 3 November, 2020) ... 99
6.4 Post-Election Period (November 4, 2020 - January 8, 2021) ... 103
6.5 Mentions ... 106
6.6 Quotes ... 109
6.7 Hyperlinks ... 110
6.8 Hashtags ... 111
7 Discussion ... 113
7.1 Denial ... 113
7.2 Downplaying the Threat ... 119
7.3 The Chinese Virus ... 121
7.4 Blame Game ... 123
7.5 Pandemic Politics ... 124
7.6 Limitations and Future Work ... 127
8 References ... 129
9 Appendix ... 186

# 1 Introduction

On the 11th of February 2020, the World Health Organization (WHO) introduced the term COVID-19 for the first time to describe the disease caused by the novel coronavirus SARS-CoV2. One month later, in light of the increasing number of infections and deaths worldwide, it characterized the virus outbreak as a pandemic thereby recognizing it as the worst public health crisis since the Spanish flu outbreak in 1918 (Barro et al., 2020).

The COVID-19 pandemic is not the first pandemic in history and it certainly will not be the last (Adhanom Ghebreyesus, 2020, December 27). However, history will mark the COVID-19 pandemic as the first of its kind to be accompanied by the internet, the web and digital media technologies (Okano-Heijmans, 2020). Search engines and social media platforms are being used on a massive scale by all members of the public as well as governments, companies, political elites, medical staff and health organizations (Vargo et al., 2020). More than 60% of the world's population are active internet users with approximately 4 billion people worldwide using social media on an average of 15% of their day time (Hootsuite & We Are Social, 2020, October 27). Consequently, since the beginning of the COVID-19 pandemic, a huge amount of unprecedented and false information has been circulating both online and offline about COVID-19. As early as February 2020, the World Health Organization described the situation as an "infodemic" (Thomas, 2020). At the same time, pandemic countermeasures, such as social distancing and lockdowns, have pushed more people to go online with almost all of the world's top social media platforms reporting strong audience growth in the third quarter of 2020 (Hootsuite & We Are Social, 2020, October 27). Twitter in particular gained around 27 million new users within only three months, from July to September 2020 (Hootsuite & We Are Social, 2020). At the same time, a significant increase in the number of followers on many state leaders' Twitter accounts was documented in March 2020 (Haman, 2020).

While there are plenty of reasons to be thankful for online technologies that have kept this huge amount of people around the world connected and informed, the role social media platforms play in amplifying rumors, increasing stigmatization, hate speech and hostility, as well as spreading conspiracy theories and personal agendas, cannot be overlooked (WHO 2020a; Eysenbach, 2020; Cinelli et al., 2020; Nielsen et al., 2020; Bavel et al., 2020). As Solomon et al. (2020, p.1806) put it, the "infodemic" the world has been experiencing since the emergence of the novel coronavirus, is, in itself, another "contagious disease infecting our information culture", which has turned the health crisis into the first "social media pandemic" in history (Guynn, 2020, March 12). Therefore, it seems more pertinent than ever to take a look at what and how information is being spread online, especially by the political elite who are considered to be the most influential actors in shaping the public opinion (Entman, 2003; Entman & Usher, 2018).

Twitter, a microblogging and social media platform, has around 350 million monthly registered users accounting for approximately 500 million tweets sent per day (Hootsuite & We Are Social, 2020, October 27; Omnicore, 2020, October 28). Three times as many people visit the platform without logging in, and since tweets are publicly available to all internet users these visitors take a more passive role and mostly treat the platform as a news website (Kemp, 2020). In the US, one in five adults say they use Twitter, and around 71% said they use it as a news source. Even before the pandemic no other social media platform played a more prominent role in the medical world than Twitter; the emergence of the virus has intensified its use for sharing and discussing medical information even by medical staff (Rosenberg et. al., 2020). It has also been extensively utilized by world leaders, especially by the 45th US President Donald Trump, as a tool of addressing the public directly (Rufai & Bunce, 2020). No other world leader has managed to steer professional media news coverage with his/her tweeting activity as Trump (Chadwick, 2017). During his presidency (January 2017-January 2021), Donald Trump's tweets continuously occupied and influenced news headlines worldwide, supported by his follower's engagement as much as his critics, thanks to the attention-based algorithms of the platform (Wells et al., 2020).

This increasing interdependence between traditional media and new digital media, as well as the continuously growing reliance on social media platforms as communication tools, whether by citizens or world leaders, is profoundly impacting "the construction of social perceptions and the framing of narratives". As a result, it is influencing "policy-making, political communication, as well as the evolution of public debate" (Cinelli at el., 2020, p.2). With this in mind, the goal of this paper is to provide an analysis of Trump's tweeting activity about the pandemic through a careful examination of his choice of words and construction of meaning around the issue, with the help of qualitative framing analysis. To achieve this goal, Trump's tweets concerning the COVID-19 pandemic from its early beginning until the suspension of his Twitter account on January 8, 2021 will be analyzed.

## 2 Relevance and Background

In a survey conducted by Nielsen et al., (2020), 54% of Americans said they rely on news organizations for information about the coronavirus while nearly as many people (49%) named the national government and politicians as their main source of information. The Pew Research Center (2020, April 29), found that 31% of Americans identified Trump and his task force as a major source for news about COVID-19, while 36% said they served as a minor source. The themes and dimensions of the pandemic focused on by this group varied from those focused on by participants who identified alternative main sources, such as the media outlets and health organizations. For example, people who mostly acquired their information from Trump and his task force were more interested in the economic impact of the pandemic than any other related issues. They were also more likely to downplay the pandemic and its effects (PEW, 2020, April 29). Moreover, those who identified Trump and his task force as their main source of information were more likely to believe in chloroquine and anti-malaria drugs such as hydroxychloroquine as treatments for the virus (PEW center, 2020, May 20). The drug was repeatedly advertised for by Trump, despite insufficient evidence about its ramifications (Solender, 2020, May 22). In a retweet from July 2020, Trump, referring to Hydroxychloroquine, even claimed that the drug can cure the coronavirus: "Covid has a cure. America wake up." (NBCNews, 2020). Twitter deleted the retweet shortly after its publication while scientific studies confirmed a lack of evidence for its efficiency leading the US Food and Drug Administration (FDA) to caution against its use outside of medical trials and hospitals (Jorge, 2020; FDA, 2020, April 24). Nevertheless, some countries, including the US, reported a sudden increase in its demand while some witnessed a spike in patients with chloroquine overdose (The Wall Street Journal, 2020, March 23; Forbes, 2020, April 9). Considering that frames are understood as major themes in a communicating text indicating how to think about a certain issue by stressing on different aspects, interpretations or solutions that might appear of less importance within another frame (Entman, 1993), these statistics might serve as an example of how framing patterns influence the public's behavior. This also aligns with Baker & Oneal's (2001, p. 682) assertion that "the public does not rally in response to crises in and of themselves, but rather to the president's handling and presentation of events".

Hence, the role of presidential leadership during a crisis becomes more important and influential than ever (Rutledge, 2020). However, Trump and his administration's response to the pandemic has been heavily criticized by scientists and political leaders for being slow, misleading, politicized, dismissive of science and expert opinions, and continuously undermining the pandemic's threat (Rutledge, 2020; Ladkin, 2020). According to the US House of Representatives Select Subcommittee on the Coronavirus Crisis (2020, p. 1) the Trump administration was "engaged in a persistent pattern of political interference—repeatedly overruling and sidelining top scientists and undermining Americans' health to advance the President's partisan agenda". A study conducted by the National Center for Disaster Preparedness at Columbia University found that, "at least 130,000 deaths and perhaps as many as 210,000 could have been avoided with earlier policy interventions and more robust federal coordination and leadership" (Redlener et al., 2020, p. 2). Similarly, Pei et al. (2020) concluded that if the

US had begun implementing control measures, such as social distancing and personal contact restrictions, one to two weeks earlier than it did, around 35,000 of the lives lost between 15, March and May 3, 2020 could have been saved and at least 600,000 infection cases prevented. Around that time, Trump was advocating for the exact opposite: to roll back state-issued social distancing restrictions and stay-at-home orders due to his main concern of saving the economy and reopening the market (Haberman, 2020, April 20; Shear & Mervosh, April 29). Trump also encouraged groups protesting against social distancing measures in states led by democratic governors such as Michigan, Minnesota and Virginia to "liberate" themselves from state-imposed restrictions (Graham et al., 2020). Despite many protesters' failure to keep social distance and wear masks, Trump described protesters as "very responsible people" who received "too tough" treatment from their local government (Hatmaker, 2020, April 17; Shear & Mervosh, April 29).

Drawing upon the interactionist theory of foundation-based moral behavior theory, Graham et al. (2020) explored participants intentions behind defying social distancing and were thereby able to provide more empirically-based evidence of Trump's effect on people's behavior. They found that people who showed higher levels of faith in Trump were more likely to express willingness to disobey social distancing measures, break stay-at-home roles and go to social events. "In fact, they are more likely to say they will do these things even if they have symptoms." (Graham et al., 2020, p. 12). Similarly, Deslatte (2020, p. 5) tested, in an artifactual survey experiment, the effects of a pro-economy frame - similar to the one predominantly adapted by Trump - on participants' willingness to take trips to the store to buy just one item despite knowing that stores "have been busier than usual, making it difficult to practice social distancing" vs. a pro-public health frame resembling the one usually adapted by scientists and experts. The results show that exposure to messages containing a pro-economy frame had a negative effect on participants, making them more willing to take unnecessary trips to the stores. Exposure to messages carrying a pro-public health frame resulted in a more positive effect in terms of adherence to social distancing measures. Interestingly, the study also reflects how the messenger persona shapes the public's behavior as participants' answers varied based on who they were told was the source. There was a "99.9% chance of a positive framing effect when the President is the messenger" of a text carrying a pro-public health frame (Deslatte, 2020, p. 8). This is the highest positive effect documented compared to the CDC, local government officials, or university experts as messengers of the same frame. "Conversely, when federal messengers - irrespective of their elected or administrative roles - present pro-economic frames, they are more likely to have a negative effect on social-distancing preferences" (Deslatte, 2020, p. 8). These findings beg the question of what could have happened if Trump's communication had been dominated by a pro-public health frame?

However, in reality Trump showed no interest in adopting such a frame and clearly expressed his refusal to fully align his policies with experts' recommendations at the cost of the economy (Tollefson, 2020, October 5). "If I listened totally to the scientists, we would right now have a country that would be in a massive depression instead — we're like a rocket ship.", he stated during a rally in Carson City, Nevada (Trump, 2020, October 19).

As a result, statistics show that trust in scientists in the US is increasingly turning into a partisan issue with 62% of left-leaning Americans saying they have a lot of trust in scientists compared to only 20% of those on the right (Funk et al., 2020, September 29). The US House of Representative's Select Subcommittee on the Coronavirus found that health experts were attacked and undermined by Trump and his administration at least 47 times between February and September 2020. This number only refers to active administrative interventions in the nation's public health response "through direct executive action or public or private pressure" excluding instances in which "Trump or his appointees downplayed the danger of the virus to the public, made false and misleading statements about the science, and misstated key facts about the Administration's response" (Select Subcommittee on the Coronavirus, 2020, October 2). In regard to misleading information, Trump was according to Evanega et al. (2020, p. 7) "likely the largest driver of the COVID-19 misinformation 'infodemic'". Around 38% of all articles containing misinformation published between January and May 2020 by English-speaking mainstream media outlets from all over the world mentioned Trump. Moreover, Trump accounted for major spikes in misinformation about "miracle cures", through his questioning of the possibility of injecting disinfection material in the body and his advocacy for hydroxychloroquine (Evanega et al. 2020, p. 7).

Trump has also failed to align his lexical choices to scientific terms in communication about the pandemic (Malouf, 2020), even though the interdependence of language, stigma, discrimination, xenophobia and public panic has continuously been highlighted by media and public health scholars (Sontag, 2001). Lessons from history show that ethnically-focused terms lead to negative effects on related communities. For example, during the H1N1 Flu outbreak in 2009-2010, the US media contributed to the stigmatization of Mexican people and those of Latin American descent, as news reports alleged the virus originated from Mexican pig farms (McCauley et al., 2013). A similar pattern of stigmatization has been growing since the emergence of COVID-19 in countries all over the world to which various public actors such as political leaders, journalists as well as individuals have actively contributed (Villa et al., 2020). Again, Trump has been a key protagonist in this regard, through the use of terms like the "China virus", the "Wuhan virus", "Chinese virus, "kung flu" and the "China plague" (Villa et al., 2020; Chang et al., 2021, March 12). Such words were used by several attackers during hate crimes against people from Asian descent in the US. For example, Denny Kim, a US Air Force veteran was personally called names such as a "Chinese virus" and "Ching Chong" while being beaten up by two attackers in Los Angeles on February 16, 2021 (McCloskey, 2021, February 25), as was an Asian American woman who was spit on and referred to as a "Chinese virus" while carrying her baby in Queens, New York City (Lenthang, 2021, March 11). The WHO predicted such a negative impact from early stages of the outbreak, and even before that, based on previous experience of health crises that were linked to geographical areas such as the Middle East Respiratory Syndrome, the Spanish Flu and the Rift Valley fever (WHO, 2015, May 8). Thus, it issued a guide on preventing and addressing social stigma in February 2020, pledging to call the virus by its scientific name only and under no circumstances by its place of origin. The organization also raised concern about how the negative usage of language plays a major role in how infected individuals and their families, as well as Asian communities are perceived and treated (WHO, 2020b).

Indeed, statistics show increasing impact on Asian communities. Many countries have reported an increase in verbal and physical attacks against people of Asian descent, while some stores in Italy even put up signs to prohibit "all people coming from China" from entering (The Guardian, 2020). The US, in particular, has been witnessing a surge in anti-Asian sentiment and attacks, some of which even rose to the level of hate crimes (Avlon, 2021, March 18). To clarify, the Federal Bureau of Investigation (FBI) defines a hate crime as any "criminal offense against a person or property motivated in whole or in part by an offender's bias against a race, religion, disability, sexual orientation, ethnicity, gender, or gender identity." (FBI, n.d.). Hate crimes could also come as a result of stigmatization since the term encompasses the convergence of the following: (1) distinguishing and labeling people based on human differences; (2) "dominant cultural beliefs linking labeled persons to undesirable characteristics" and people associating human differences with negative stereotypes and attributions; (3) such "social labels connote a separation of 'us' from 'them'" (Link and Phelan, 2001, p. 370); and (4) "labeled persons experience status loss and discrimination that lead to unequal outcomes." (Link and Phelan, 2001, p. 367). Stigmatization "is entirely contingent on access to social, economic, and political power" that allow for the abovementioned behaviors to happen leading to "execution of disapproval, rejection, exclusion, and discrimination" of certain people or groups (Link and Phelan, 2001, p. 367). The term xenophobia on the other hand, has been historically used to refer to fear of people who are perceived as not native to the land or dominant culture (Wimmer, 1997). However, more recently, the term is being linked to "ethnocentrism, which is characterized by the attitude that one's own group or culture is superior to others" and has therefore come to be used to denote anti-immigrant prejudice including any type of 'us' vs 'them' rhetoric (Yakushko, 2009, p. 44). In a joint publication the International Labour Office (ILO), International Organization for Migration (IOM), and Office of the United Nations High Commissioner for Human Rights (OHCHR) define xenophobia as any "prejudices and behavior that reject, exclude and often vilify persons, based on the perception that they are outsiders or foreigners to the community, society or national identity" (ILO et al., 2001, p. 1).

Stop Asian American and Pacific Islander (AAPI) is a non-profit organization formed by the Asian Pacific Planning and Policy Council (A3PCON), Chinese for Affirmative Action (CAA), and the Asian American Studies Department of San Francisco State University as a response to the rise of anti-Asian American violence amid the COVID-19 pandemic. Between March 2020 and February 2021, they have documented 3,795 such discriminatory incidents across the US. Of these incidents, 68.1% were verbal harassments while 11.1% were physical assaults (Jeung et al., 2021, March 16). Similarly, by analyzing preliminary data released by 16 police departments of America's largest cities, the Center for the Study of Hate and Extremism at California State University revealed a 149% increase in anti-Asian hate crimes in the US during

2020 (CSUSB, 2021, March 2). In New York city alone, out of the 29 crimes against people from Asian descent that occurred in 2020, 24 had clear "coronavirus motivations" according to the city's police department (Sturla et al., 2021, February 27).

Still, experts believe that these numbers reflect a "tiny fraction of the total" (Thorbecke, 2020, February 25). Anti-Asian hate crime data in the US remains "unreliable and underreported" (Krishnakumar, 2021, March 18): law enforcement agencies in the country are not obliged to report hate crimes data to the FBI and often fails to do so. In turn, distrust in governmental agencies on the part of Asian American communities leads victims from these communities to refrain from reporting (Krishnakumar, 2021, March 18). Meanwhile, survey data published by the PEW research center in July 2020 confirms that Asian American communities feel affected by the pandemic, as 31% of participants of Asian descent reported they had been victims of slurs or jokes in relation to their race or ethnicity since the beginning of the outbreak, while 26% admitted that they "feared someone might threaten or physically attack them" (Ruiz et al., 2020, July 1).

According to the WHO, "governments, citizens, media, key influencers and communities have an important role to play in preventing and stopping stigma surrounding people from China and Asia in general" (WHO, 2020b, p. 3) - a role Trump and his administration has been continuously criticized for failing to uphold. In a memorandum published only six days after Joe Biden was sworn in as a President, Biden wrote: "The Federal Government must recognize that it has played a role in furthering these xenophobic sentiments through the actions of political leaders, including references to the COVID-19 pandemic by the geographic location of its origin." (Biden, 2021, January 26). Hswen et al., (2021) provide empirical evidence of this effect as their study shows a huge rise (19 462.6%) in the number of Tweets using the #chinesevirus hashtag during the week following March 16, 2020, the day Trump published his first tweet with reference to the coronavirus as the "Chinese virus", as compared to the previous week. The hashtag #chinesevirus thereby surpassed the number of tweets using the more neutral hashtag #covid19 which had been the predominant term before March 16, 2020. However, what is even more alarming is the significant rise in the appearance of other anti-Asian hashtags such as #bateatingchinese, #disgustingchinese and #makethecommiechinesepay in the week after the President's tweet. Nonetheless, it should be noted that 20% of hashtags associated with the #covid19 hashtag also contained anti-Asian sentiment, while approximately half of those accompanied by #chinesevirus did so. Thus, the study findings indicate "a rise in prejudicial language following some of the president's tweets" and reflect how "racist attitudes may be reinforced by institutional support" (Hswen et al., p. e5-e6).

Based on observing the above-mentioned developments, this paper was initiated to offer a contribution to the scholarly work aimed at understanding Trump's communication style, particularly on Twitter, which until the suspension of his account on January 8, 2021 functioned as his "biggest political megaphone" (Gambino, 2021, January 9). More specifically, it is an attempt to examine how the platform was used as a tool of communication in response to the pandemic by the highest member of the US political elite. With this in mind, the goal of this thesis will be to explore what framing patterns dominated Trump's tweets about the COVID-19 pandemic. What aspects of the pandemic did Trump focus on? How did Trump use Twitter to frame the virus, specify causes of the pandemic, convey related moral assessments and endorse remedies (Entman, 1993)? What interpretation do his lexical choices put forward and what type of language was used? To what extent does the language used in tweets reinforce xenophobia and fear? What type of information sources did he rely on? Did the tweets contain blaming messages and who was to blame? What solutions were offered? And What appeals were made to the public?

Thus, the main research question that will guide this paper is: What framing patterns dominated Trump's tweeting activity about COVID-19?

# 3 Framing Theory

When a message is sent out to the public what matters most is not only what is said but how it is said along with what is not being said (Heck, 1987; Entman 1993; Gamson & Modigliani, 1989). This process of intentionally highlighting and accentuating certain aspects in a communicating text, while negating the salience of other aspects in order to shape the recipients' understanding of an issue is referred to within the field of communication studies as framing (Entman, 1993; D'Angelo, 2002). The main premise of the concept is that an issue can be viewed and presented from various perspectives, thereby influencing the recipients' opinion formation, subsequent action and relevant issue evaluation (Chong & Druckman, 2007a). Metaphorically speaking, one could think of frames as the lenses through which we view, filter and make sense of our world and daily experiences, while framing is the process used to intentionally direct, reorient or limit the perspective of these lenses towards certain positions or worldviews (Druckman 2007; Entman 1993; Tuchman, 1978).

Since the postulation of the concept in psychological and sociological studies during the mid 70s, the concept has been widely used and adapted within various disciplines including sociological, political, economic and linguistic research fields, as well as in communications and media studies (Van Gorp, 2007). As a result, multiple conceptual and operational definitions of frames and framing have arisen, leading Entman (1993, p. 51) to characterize the framing research field as a "fractured paradigm" (see also, D'Angelo, 2002; D'Angelo et. al., 2019; de Vreese, 2012; Borah, 2011). Some scholars consider this polarization as a weakness of the framing research paradigm and call for a unified theoretical framework (Cacciatore et al., 2016) as well as methodological approach (Matthes & Kohring, 2008). Krippendorff (2017) has even called for an entire abandonment of the concept. According to D'Angelo (2002, p. 871) "there is not, nor should there be, a single paradigm of framing" as its "[t]heoretical and paradigmatic diversity has led to a comprehensive view of the framing process" thereby "harnessing the power of communication's paradigms", building extensive knowledge about a "complex process" (D'Angelo, 2002, p. 883) and allowing room for more creativity (Hertog & Mcleod, 2001). In fact, more recently D'Angelo (2019, p. 14) argued that "[t]he 'fractured' nature of framing research is its strength" adding that "the study of framing is itself an enterprise pushing the boundaries of knowledge about societies, media, and citizens."(D'Angelo, 2019, p, 17). Lule (2019) agrees with D'Angelo (2019) as he denies notions to abandon or go beyond framing research and instead asserts: "Let a thousand framers frame" (Lule, 2020, p. 17). Nonetheless, while calling for the "return of the repressed" referring to the need to bring back language into the focus of framing in media studies (Lule, 2019, p. 19). As follows, Lule (2019) also highlighted the need to conduct more qualitative studies in which most attention is given to interpreting language beyond mere quantitative coding of texts with the help of algorithms. Similarly, de Vreese (2012, p. 367) favors maintaining a "broad and inclusive definition of frames" instead of limiting the broad applicability of the concept to one "golden, definitive [and] standard definition". However, he underlines the importance of establishing a solid theoretical and methodological basis within each individual framing study (de Vreese, 2012, p. 367).

For this reason, this chapter seeks to unravel what is meant by frames and framing within the scope of this study. At the beginning, the origins of the term will be tracked down taking into consideration Borah's (2011, p. 255) assertion that "although frames in communication and their influence on the audience are equally important, understanding the origin of the frames is essential for a more complete picture of framing". Entman (1993, p. 52) identifies four locations in which frames could be found during communication processes; First, at the communicator's level referring to the individual's frame in thought or their "schemata of interpretation" (see also, Goffman, 1974, p. 21) that consciously or unconsciously guides and influence how frames appear in the second location which is the communicating text. In texts, frames are manifested in the use of language and choice of words found within it such as "the presence or absence of certain keywords, stock phrases, stereotyped images, sources of information, and sentences that provide thematically reinforcing clusters of facts or judgments." (Entman 1993, p. 52). The third location is on the recipient's cognitive level, given that each individual mental structure is different and thereby also their interaction with and interpretation of the frames found in a communicating text. The fourth location listed by Entman (1993, p. 52) refers to the dominant culture as it represents a source of "commonly invoked frames" that are a result of as well as influencers of other frames found in all mentioned locations.

The existence of frames in the first two locations; mind and text, are the cause of what is referred to as "[T]he dual nature of framing research" (Borah, 2011, p. 249). Although this paper is focused only on identifying frames located in text, which is in this case represented in tweets, the duality of framing research will be illustrated within the following chapter to provide a comprehensive understanding of what framing research entails and to demonstrate why the second location was chosen for the purposes of this study. Moreover, taking into consideration, Lule's (2019, p. 19) call for the "return of the repressed" the role language plays in framing and political communication will also be discussed.

### 3.1 Origins

The term frame was first articulated by Bateson in *The Message: This is Play*, a presentation given in 1956 at the Macy Conference on Small Groups (Steier, 2013). However, Bateson's later more developed work A theory of play and fantasy, published in 1972, is usually identified in research as the urtext of the term (Hallahan, 1999; Van Hulst & Yanow, 2016). Bateson (1972) introduced frames as cognitive structures that enable humans to draw the boundaries of a social encounter through signaling out cues, whether verbal or non-verbal, to bring common interpretation of the situation at hand to mind. To clarify, cognition is defined as "our faculty of knowing and understanding something in a specific way and how we base our behaviour and thinking on such knowledge" (Fourie 2001, p. 298). In this sense, frames guide how the human mind makes sense of its surroundings (Bateson, 1972; Goffman, 1975).

During an observation made at the Zoo, Bateson noted that a bite given from one monkey to the other did not trigger a fight between the two counterparts but rather a playful encounter although a bite could be just as well be interpreted as a sign of hostility. Thus, he concluded that the two monkeys must have shared some kind of "metacommunication" that is "messages about the messages" (Fisher, p. 295). These communication cues, according to Bateson, enabled both actors to interpret the bite within what he referred to as the "This is play" frame; "The playful nip denotes the bite, but it does not denote what would be denoted by the bite" (Bateson, 1972, p. 180). In other words, the monkeys must have shared some signals that triggered a common mood of play in which the bite is not understood as a sign of fighting (Bateson, 1972).

Humans, Bateson argues, can similarly communicate on various levels of abstraction; it is the presence of different types of psychological frames used to interpret the same communication clue that allows the human mind to distinguish between the different levels of meaning. Therefore, Bateson (1972) defined a frame as "a certain set of rules for the making and understanding of messages" (Bateson, 1972, p. 191). In the same manner in which a physical picture frame organizes a viewer's perception by bordering elements within it thereby signaling a certain type of connection bonding the elements together, psychological frames organize how the mind decodes and evaluates messages by signaling which communicative clues are mutually relevant within the given context and should therefore be focused on. Herewith, frames define a "system of relationships between massages" (Bateson, 1972, p. 190). However, this inclusive function of frames automatically gives them an exclusive function as well; given that they isolate whatever lies beyond the frame's borders indicating what should in return be ignored. "Attend to what is within and do not attend to what is outside" (Bateson, 1972, p. 187). Hence, a frame does not only define what the message is but also what it is not. Or as Houseman (2012, p.1) puts it through frames a "particular kind of social action is defined by the manner in which it is distinguished". Going back to Bateson's example this would mean that the "This is play" frame also holds within it a this is "not combat" frame (Bateson, 1972, p. 179). For this reason, it is evident to recognize the recursive and possibly paradoxical relationship between meaning and context (Bateson, 1972). And it is because of the different mental structures framing can shape, that humans are able to draw lines between the relevant and irrelevant and choose from different lines of logical thinking needed to understand the meaning of messages within their context and sometimes beyond their donative level; the literal meaning of words (Bateson, 1972).

Sociologist Ervin Goffman (1974) credited Bateson for coining the term. However, he adapted it to the sociological field by offering a more detailed clarification of framing as a process of constructing meaning and guiding social action; "[D]efinitions of a situation are built up in accordance with principles of organization which govern events [...] and our subjective involvement in them" (Goffman, 1974, p. 10). He argued that although individuals might not always be able to identify what frames they employ to make sense of the world around them, they use framing to give answers to the question: "What is going on here?" (Goffman, 1974, p. 21). Thereby, frames function as "schemata of interpretations" that help "locate, perceive, identify, and label" social events that would otherwise remain a countless number of meaningless messages (Goffman, 1974, p. 21). As a result, each individual constructs their own image of reality based on personal experiences which in return also guides people's action. Senge (1990) would refer to this image as a personal "mental model" which is the individual's picture of how the world works. Hence, frames were seen as cognitive, interactive and context related mental models consistent with Aronsson's description of frames as "the conditions of social interaction" (Aronsson, 2002, p. 68).

Although, according to Reese et. al. (2003, p. 11), frames are "persistent over time" this does not mean that they are entirely static. Frames may vary and evolve over time and space with the evolution of different social, political as well as cultural ideas and developments (Hallahan, 1999). As Edelman (1993, p. 332) puts it, "The social world is [...] a kaleidoscope of potential realities, any of which can be readily evoked by altering the way in which observations are framed and categorized". Frames are, however, socially constructed and shared, according to Goffman (1974) who argued that societies produce common understandings of issues from which collective primary frameworks rooted in culture emerge. Given that individuals as members of a society will be repeatedly exposed to a certain set of socially shared frames, they consequently become more dominant by being more accessible, retrievable and available in memory to be used as the common frames of reference for forming "judgments, opinions and decisions" (Iyengar, 199, p. 2). This has led Entman (1993, p. 52) to argue that culture itself could be defined as "the empirically demonstrable set of common frames exhibited in the discourse and thinking of most people in a social grouping."

### 3.2 The Power of a Communicating Text

Building on Goffman's work, Tuchman (1978) and Gitlin (1980) main argument was if frames are socially constructed, then the question that arises is who drives and influences the social construction process from which primary frameworks of societies emerge? Both Tuchman (1978) and Gitlin (1980) identified news organizations as primary sources and influential agents in constructing social reality. In the news, the parameters "in which citizens discuss public events" are set (Tuchman, 1978, p. IV). This is done through using frames as tools "to process large amounts of information quickly and routinely package the information for efficient relay to the [...] audiences" (Gitlin, 1980, p. 7). While Gitlin (1980, p. 7) recognized the original meaning of frames offered by Bateson (1972) and Goffman (1974) by stating first that news frames are "persistent patterns of cognition", he went further to highlight how exactly frames come to stand and are then communicated to audiences by stating that they are also "principles of selection, emphasis and presentation composed of little tacit theories about what exists, what happens, and what matters". As follows, he concluded that frames get picked up by journalists as tools that help organize their world by enabling the reduction and classification of the big burden and quick flow of information they face in their routinized newsrooms. However, the journalist's choice of frames usually differs based on the type of organization in which a journalist works, their national context, political ideology as well as information sources and resources (Tuchman, 1978; Gitlin, 1980; Pan and Kosicki, 1993; Snow et al., 2007; Van Gorp, 2010). As such, media framing processes were seen as "outcomes of social interactions between political and media actors and environments that are for the greater part routinized and tapping into common sense." (Vliegenthart & van Zoonen, 2011, p. 107). Therefore, scholars within the critical research paradigm of framing argue that frames that align with the "perspective of values held by political and economic elites" are more likely to be picked up by journalists and subsequently dominate news and thereby also audiences (D'Angelo 2020, p. 876; see also, Entman, 1991; Solomon 1992).

In consequence, the three keywords "selection, emphasis and presentation" mentioned by Gitlin's (1980, p. 7) have since then caused a shift in framing research from looking at frames as "schemata of interpretation" that exists in people's mind to looking at how a certain "schemata of interpretation" regarding an issue becomes more available, accessible and applicable to the public. Especially through investigating how different social actors such as politicians, governmental and non-governmental organizations as well as social movements actively frame public issues (Snow et al, 1986; Borah, 2011). Consequently, tapping into the question of; How do certain schemata of interpretation become more dominant than others? (Gamson & Modigliani, 1989; Entman, 1993). And how do media, political and advocacy actors try to actively "polish their images and frame debates over public policies" thereby raising the question on the other hand, of how audiences make sense of and interact with such polished frames based on their existing cognitive knowledge? (Pan & Kosicki, 1993, p. 55).

Thus clearly, if frames do not first exist, whether consciously or unconsciously, in an individual's mind as sense-making tools, filtering out relevant thoughts from irrelevant ones, then they certainly could not be exerted upon or communicated to others. Also, without the existence of at least one frame in thought, citizens would not be able to make sense of media and political communication including the frames they carry (Kinder & Sanders, 1996). Therefore, while recognizing the role of frames as "internal structures of the mind" (Kinder & Sanders, 1990, p. 47) and "prior knowledge" used to organize thought and process information as suggested by scholars within the cognitive research paradigm of framing (D'Angelo, 2002, p. 873), this paper is more concerned with doing framing research in line with Entman's suggestion "as a way to describe the power of a communicating text" and "luminate the precise way in which influence over a human conscious-ness is exerted by the transfer (or communication) of information from one location-such as a speech, utterance, news report, or novel-to that consciousness." (Entman 1993, p. 51-52).

### 3.3 Function of Frames

Consequently, speaking of frames within the scope of this paper refers to the "result of the framing process" as suggested by Matthes (2011, p. 252) while framing is "an active process of creating, selecting and shaping the frames." However, it is important to clarify that frames are "not singular persuasive messages or assertions" but rather "always refer to a pattern involving issue interpretation, attribution, and evaluation" (Matthes, 2011, p. 252.). They have an organizational and structural function connecting different elements within a communicating text together, thereby ideally feeding into a consistent pattern of interpretation in line with Gamson & Modigliani (1989, p. 3) definition of a frame as an "interpretive package" (see also, Reese, 2007). Similarly, Pan and Kosicki (1993) suggest thinking of frames as themes that emerge as a result of a "system of organized signifying elements that both indicate the advocacy of certain ideas and provide devices to encourage certain kinds of audience processing of the texts." (Pan & Kosicki, p. 55).

So far, we have established that the framing process involves inclusion and exclusion of certain aspects in the communication process as well as emphasis put on certain aspects which is what Entman (1993, p. 52) calls "salience" defined as "making a piece of information more noticeable, meaningful, or memorable to audiences". These processes of selecting and saliencing lie at the core of one of the most cited and widely accepted definitions of framing (David et al., 2011; Borah, 2011) offered by Entman (1993, p. 52) who writes:

> To frame is to select some aspects of a perceived reality and make them more salient in a communicating text, in such a way as to promote a particular problem definition, causal interpretation, moral evaluation, and/or treatment recommendation for the item described.

According to Entman (2003), problem definition constitutes one of the two most important functions of frames alongside treatment recommendation as it relates to presenting the core issue at hand indicating what should be focused on, its causes, benefits, related actors, main keywords and arguments, possibly also consequences and ramifications. The problem tends to be outlined in relation to dominant and shared cultural values since these determine how much a frame resonates within the public discourse (Entman, 1993; Van Gorp, 2007). Therefore, "defining the problem often virtually predetermines the rest of the frame" (Entman, 2003, p. 417-418) which is why Gamson and Modigliani (1989, p.3) argue that at the core of frames lies a "central organizing idea". The proposed solutions and strategies are also crucial since they usually require action. Herewith, guiding and possibly influencing subsequent decision-making processes on various levels.

In the case of COVID-19 pandemic, for example, suggesting wearing masks or taking certain medication gives the public suggestions on how to deal with or protect themselves from the spread of COVID-19 which might have a direct impact on their safety or lives. As Entman (1993, p. 54) puts it a "frame determines whether most people notice and how they understand and remember a problem, as well as how they evaluate and choose to act upon it." The fourth above mentioned function is especially critical given that treatment recommendation might, in some cases, especially within strategic political communication, be advocating and mobilizing for the endorsement of or opposition to actual governmental policies and actions (Entman, 1993). In addition, one of the main functions of frames is to highlight and bring a certain type of interpretation regarding the problem definition closer to the recipients' minds making the frame more available and accessible for application. Interpretations often entail identifying who is to be held responsible or what the causes are. Moral judgments are often based on the perceived benefits and risks of an issue thus they are usually gradual and reflect to which degree an issue is negatively or positively viewed although it could also be ambivalent (Entman, 1993, 2003, 2004).

Another important part of the framing processes is repetition which plays a role in influencing how framing patterns arise and impact audiences (Chong & Druckman, 2007; Entman, 2003). For example, Matthes (2008) concluded that only frames that appear frequently in news texts are likely to have an impact on recipients. Thus, repetition in communication “leads to a higher and more constant level of accessibility, which in turn increases the applicability of a framed message” (de Vreese, 2012, p. 370). Matthes (2011, p. 252) similarly argues that “[f]rames exert their power by repeatedly invoking the same pattern of consistent frame elements giving citizens a chance to notice, understand, and store the mental association for future applications." President Bush and his administration’s framing patterns in communication following the September 11 attacks in 2001 serve as an example according to Entman (2003, p. 416), who argued that the continuous repetition of the same war-related terminology such as “war act” and “evil enemy”, embedded the terms in US media and public discourse making it almost impossible to define the situation or discuss its causes and treatments apart from a certain association to the war frame.

Moreover, salience could also be achieved through the intentional instrumentalization of certain keywords, stock- and catchphrases, figurative language as well as the use of information linkage in close connection to an existing schemata of interpretation in the recipients’ belief system and culture such as stereotypes and religious or historical exemplars (Gitlin, 1980; Entman, 1993). Culturally resonating elements help make a frame more “noticeable, understandable, memorable and emotionally charged” for the recipients (Entman, 2003, p. 417). The more inclusive a frame of elements that resonate with the recipients’ culture, the more likely their influence on the recipients. Therefore, Entman (2003, p, 417) highlights that the four aforementioned framing functions are usually achieved “in a kind of cultural logic, serving each other, with the connections cemented more by custom and convention than by principles of valid reasoning or syllogistic logic." (Entman, 2003, p. 417)

### 3.4 Emphasis vs. Equivalence Framing

In light of more recent attempts to clarify conceptual definitions of frames it should be said that this paper is concerned with analyzing emphasis framing also referred to as issue framing rather than equivalence framing (Cacciatore et al., 2016; Chong & Druckman 2007a; Druckman 2001). Cacciatore et al. (2016) call for a strict differentiation between the two, arguing that equivalence framing refers to altering or manipulating the demonstration of factually and logically equal information thereby leading to a change in the recipient's choice or policy preferences. This type of framing usually involves "casting the same information in either a positive or negative light" (Druckman 2004, p. 671). For example, issues could be framed of either having a 90% success rate vs. a 10% failure rate without any actual change taken on the facts, content or outcomes of the two options (Druckman, 2007a). Since the start of the COVID-19 vaccination processes, political and media actors have been defying the vaccination processes in terms of the positive percentage of people having been vaccinated e.g.: 40% of US citizens received the vaccine or by numbers e.g. 2 million people have been vaccinated (see for example Holder, 2021, February 5). The alternative equivalent frame in this case would be presenting the progress in terms of the percentage of people that have not been vaccinated e.g.: 60% of US citizens did not receive the vaccine yet. Long before the COVID-19 pandemic, Tversky and Kahneman (1981, p.453) led the way in investigating the effect of equivalency framing by creating a fictional situation of "an unusual Asian disease" outbreak that is expected to kill 600 people. After exposing participants to solutions that will eventually lead to the same results, they found that the opposing negative and positive formulations of the sentences caused a change in preference on the participants' side; A positive portrayal of the gains (lives saved) has been proven to be more persuasive than a negative portrayal of the loss (lives lost). Moreover, the authors concluded that people are less likely to take risks when their choices are presented in terms of potential gains but more likely to take risks to avoid potential losses (Tversky and Kahneman, 1981). Hence, equivalence framing, similar to emphasis framing, also rotates around shifting the recipients' focus on certain considerations. However, the main difference is that equivalency frames are employed to present "materially identical descriptions" while emphasis frames ideally focus on "qualitatively different yet potentially relevant considerations" (Chong & Druckman, 2007a). For example, when Sniderman & Theriaul (2004) asked participants; "Given the importance of free speech", would you be in favor of or against allowing a hate group to hold a political rally? 85% answered that they would be in favor. However, when the introductory sentence was intentionally replaced with words saliencing another aspect by asking the question in terms of; "Given the risk of violence", would you be in favor of or against allowing a hate group to hold a political rally? Only 45% said they would be in favor. Unlike the above-mentioned positive and negative frames of the vaccinations rate, the two free speech and public safety frames cannot logically be equated together which reflects that main difference between the two types of framing (Cacciatore et al., 2016; Chong & Druckman, 2007a).

### 3.5 Framing Effect

However, what connects the two types of framing, whether equivalence or emphasis framing, is their ability to lead to changes in preferences on the recipients' side. This change is referred to by scholars as the framing effect defined as "one in which salient attributes of a message (its organization, selection of content, or thematic structure) render particular thoughts applicable, resulting in their activation and use in evaluations" (Price et al., 1997, p. 486).

Nevertheless, this does not inherently mean that the role of existing individual schemata of interpretation in processing information offered by the media or the political elite is entirely illuminated but rather serves as a basis to "alternatively, accept, ignore and reinterpret the dominant frames offered" Neuman et al. (1992, p. 62). Salience is "a product of the interaction of texts and receivers" as Entman (1993, p. 53) puts it. An individual's prior knowledge influences how recipients make sense of information. Although the goal of a communicator may be to prevent the recipient from another schemata of interpretation, it is unlikely that they are always fully successful in achieving this goal (Van Gorp, 2007, p. 63). Several individual factors on the recipients' side may influence the degree of frame effect such as their level of education, social class and political orientation or perceived judgment of the speaker's credibility (Borah, 2011; de Vreese & Lecheler, 2012; Chong & Druckman 2007a, 2007b; Slothuus, 2008). For example, Chong and Druckman (2007b) found that people with higher levels of political interest are less likely to be affected by political framing and more likely to dismiss weak frames since they will spend more cognitive effort to vet different competitive frames in democratic environments against each other, before choosing which one is more applicable. The same goes for people with higher levels of education who are "better able to resist incongruent information and maintain alignment between their factual beliefs and predispositions" (Flynn et al., 2017, 136).

This paper is focused on understanding how meaning is constructed through framing messages on the communicators' side, therefore studying the exact mechanism of how framing effects take place falls outside the scope of this study. However, it is important to clarify that this paper does not assume a linear effect of framing taking into consideration that the framing effect occurs when ''frames in communication'' subsequently affect ''frames in thought'' and that various factors could influence this process (Chong & Druckman, 2007a, p. 109).

### 3.6 When the Power of a Communicating Text Meets the Power of the Oval Office

Thus, political communicators strategically tailor their frames in communication in a way that may best align with their audiences' existing schemata of interpretation, which are "themselves largely products of prior framing" (Entman & Usher, 2018). However, given that political competitors usually seek different strategies requiring policies that could rarely be logically equivalent, emphasis framing is more employed by political actors than equivalence framing (Slothuus & De Vreese, 2010).

For Chong (1993, p. 870), framing is the "essence of public opinion formation". Similarly, Van Gorp (2007, p. 63) argues that the ability to manipulate knowledge about the receiver's culture in favor of reaching the desired framing effects, makes frames "mechanisms of power in their own right". Political elites recognize these assertions and are aware that under competitive democratic circumstances framing is an essential tool of exercising power over the public, since power manifests itself in the ability of getting others to behave and act in line of one's own policies or desires (Nagel, 1975; Levin 2005; Entman, 2007). As a result, framing is often deployed by political actors to facilitate desirable policies to the public and/or constrain undesirable ones as well as to mobilize supporters (Slothuus & De Vreese, 2010). Edelman (1993, p. 51) argues that "authorities and pressure groups categorize beliefs in a way that marshals support and oppositions to their interest". Therefore, for D'Angelo (2019), the first conceptual salience based definition offered by Entman (1993) is insufficient to describe framing and is rather only when accompanied with Entman's latter definition in which framing is described as "the central process by which government officials and journalists exercise political power over each other and the public" (Entman, 2003, p. 417) able to reflect how "framing-building and framing-effects occur diachronically" and shed light on the role power games "cultural congruence, resonance, magnitude and network" play in the process (D'Angelo, 2019, p. 15).

### *3.6.1 Cascading Network Activation*

According to the cascading network activation model formulated by Entman (2003), the political elite sitting in Washington's White House is considered the most powerful group in spreading ideas throughout the general information system, thereby building and shaping frames of the public discourse. Above all, it is the president and his top advisors, given their administrative power, who have the greatest ability to attract attention and shape mental associations regarding issues by spreading them through the flow of political communication, followed by the non-administrative elite such as members of the congress and political experts. The third level of influence comprises traditional institutional media institutions and at the lowest level, the public (Entman, 2003). This is not to say that frames can solely be activated by powerful social actors but that their flow is easier coming down from upper levels than going up. As the metaphor used in the model's name suggests; water flows easier down a cascading waterfall than up. Thus, feedback loops do take place (Entman, 2003).

Members within each of the levels represented in the cascading model play, to a certain extent, a role in the formulation and diffusion of frames into the general information system. However, those usually require extra effort, a "pumping mechanism" as Entman (2003, p. 420) describes it, in order for their ideas or counter frames to be able to attract attention and be carried up from one level to the other. The most powerful are those frames offered by the president who is considered the highest-ranking member of the political elite in countries with a presidential system like the one in the US (Entman,

2003; Rutledge, 2020). Hence, after their activation, presidential frames travel simultaneously given that they already possess the frame success factor of prominence which "arises above all from their control over the government apparatus" and the ability to directly influence and shape "'facts on the ground'" (Entman, 2003, p. 422). They are also easily able to reach frame repetition as members of the second level such as the executive branch or ex-officials are forced to react and take position on the offered frame. Thereby, often turning it into the frame of reference on the issue at hand and to a certain degree reinforcing it (Entman, 2003; Entman & Usher, 2018). The press also contributes to this process, whether its redistribution of presidential frames is driven by its ideological and political alliances or its desire to function as watchdogs of the public interest (Bennet et al., 2005). Thus, even when the press practices criticism, by repeating the language used in the frame, the press contributes to the activation and spread of that particular frame (Entman & Usher, 2018; Lakoff, 2014).

### *3.6.2 All Thought is Physical*

This is because "all thought is physical" as professor of cognitive science and linguistics George Lakoff explains it in his book: *The all new don't think of an elephant!: Know your values and frame the debate* (Lakoff, 2014, p. 1). The way language works is through activating what is referred to in cognitive science as "neural circuits" of the brain. A lot of this activation happens unconsciously and with no possibility of consciously accessing or intervening in the process (Lakoff, 2014). In that way, language is made meaningful through "the ways those neural circuits are connected to the body and characterize embodied experience" (Lakoff, 2012, p. 773). The neural structures built allow us to make sense of abstract ideas and connect them to certain meanings. However, these are not easy to change; rather they are deeply and relatively fixed (Lakoff, 2012, 2014). This means that "[a]ll words are defined relative to conceptual frames" thus when a word is heard, its frame gets automatically activated in the brain (Lakoff, 2014, p. 2). For example, after having read the name of Lakoff's book mentioned above, it is almost impossible not to think of a bulky gray animal with long nose and floppy ears, argues the author. Hence, when a frame is being refuted its activation still occurs thereby increasing the cognitive strength of its frame-circuit (Lakoff, 2014). "In order to negate something in the brain, you have to activate it first. Then you can negate it. But when you activate it neurally, you're strengthening the neural circuitry that is being used." (Lakoff, 2017, April 18). For example, when President Nixon said "I am not a crook" in the aftermath of the watergate scandal "everybody thought about him as a crook" (Lakoff, 2014, p. 1). The same goes to repeating frames, it deepens the mental structures created by the frame and makes listeners unconsciously think of the manner in terms of the words used in the frame regardless of whether it is accompanied by criticism or not. "The more a word is heard, the more the circuit is activated and the stronger it gets, and so the easier it is to fire again" (Lakoff, 2016, July 23).

According to Lakoff, Trump understands the power of repeating words and employs it when he keeps repeating words like "Fake news" (See Meeks, 2020). As Lakoff (2016, July 23) puts it: "Trump uses your brain against you". For this reason, Lakoff continuously advises social actors who seek to practice criticism on Trump's issue framing, not to repeat or retweet his words: "When you repeat Trump, you help Trump. You do this by spreading his message wide and far" (Lakoff, 2018, May 24). This might also explain why correcting political misperceptions sometimes backfires, triggering a boomerang effect that deepens those beliefs (Nyhan & Reifler, 2010). Instead, Lakoff (2014) advocates for actively re-framing issues with the use of one's own choice of words that directly activate the frame one seeks to establish, instead of negating the other with the use of the same words. "That is what framing is about. Framing is about getting language that fits your worldview. It is not just language. The ideas are primary—and the language carries those ideas, evokes those ideas." (Lakoff, 2014, p. 2)

Nonetheless, it is worth mentioning that "there is nothing inherently superior about an applicable or strong frame other than its appeal to audiences. "Strong frames should not be confused with intellectually or morally superior arguments" (Chong & Druckman, 2007a, p. 111). Perhaps the most recent example of how influential the words used by political leaders to frame issues could be, is reflected in the storming of the Capitol Hill on January 6, 2021. Numerous journalists, world leaders and US politicians accused Trump of inciting the attacks especially through his speech shortly before the riots, in which Trump used the words "fight" or "fighting" no less than 25 times (Rupar, 2020, January 8). "We are going to have to fight much harder". "You'll never take back our country with weakness. You have to show strength. You have to be strong", are just a few examples of the narrative Trump built in his speech (Rupar, 2020, January 8). Indeed, these actions led to his impeachment by the House of Representatives for the "incitement of insurrection", making him the first US president to be subjected to impeachment twice (BBC, 2020, January 14). On the 8th of January 2020, Twitter permanently suspended his account "due to the risk of further incitement of violence" (Twitter, 2021, January 8). President elect Joe Biden said after the attacks: "the words of a President matter, no matter how good or bad that president is. At their best, the words of a president can inspire. At their worst, they can incite" (Biden, 2021, January 6). Although it is arguable how much of that is also framing done on Biden's side, his words offer a reflection of how effective presidential frames could be.

## 3.7 When the Power of a Communicating Text Meets the Power of Digital Media

### *3.7.1 The Hybrid Media System*

Recent technological advances are constantly changing the characteristic of information flow by opening new paths that make online, intersectional and quick means of communication and information gathering available to the public (Shah et al., 2017). Above all, digitalized communication methods such as social media platforms have created online public spheres in which citizens can directly address and send their messages to the political elite without the necessity of having traditional media institutions as transmitters in between (Entman & Usher, 2018). This has led to a more "decentralized, interconnected, and reciprocal" media system and a rather diffused flow of information compared to Entman's (2003) unidirectional cascade model (Meeks, 2020, p. 213). All level members within the newer system have become content creators and power has shifted towards those able to gain more attention online (Chadwick, 2017). The nature of information consumption is changed, as audience members before the rise of online media “received messages in isolation from other audience members and their responses were largely passive, with limited opportunities to provide feedback to the content creators” (Shah et al., 2017, p. 4). However, nowadays, members of all levels receive political messages as well as news coverage in an interconnected environment that enables circular feedback loops on large scales (Shah et al., 2017). As a result, the boundaries between members of the public are blurred and those between the political elite and the media “appear less permeable” (Entman & Usher, 2018, p. 7).

Chadwick (2017, xi) characterizes the current media system as “hybrid”, one in which traditional print and broadcast media function along, interact and coevolve with, as well as adapt themselves to, new digital media. The result is a more complex, coexisting and interdependent relationship between the two and a fundamental change in political communication described by Chadwick (2017, xi) as a “chaotic transition period”. Within the current media system actors “are articulated by complex and ever-evolving relationships based upon adaptation and interdependence and simultaneous concentrations and diffusions of powers" (Chadwick, 2017, p. 3). Herewith, Chadwick (2017, p. xi) highlights the existence of a blended mixture between “older and newer media logics” rather than the belief that one is taking over or replacing the other. In this case, logics stand for “technologies, genres, norms, behaviors, and organizational forms—in the reflexively connected fields of media and politics (Chadwick, 2017, p. 4). For example, traditional media has adapted itself to new digital media logics by reproducing content in different formats to fit into the nature of various social media Platforms. To post on Twitter, the content has to come in the form of 280 characters maximum, Instagram requires visual content while Facebook allows for more room to integrate older media logics on the Platform (Chadwick, 2017). At the same time, new media logics manifested in digital media platforms and search engines are granting a more inclusive and influential role in the cycle of political communication to the public as well as non-governmental organizations (Powers, 2014). Under the umbrella of the hybrid media system, ideas originating from lower levels of Entman's (2003) original cascading activation model have higher chances of being pushed up the levels to reach the political elite and onto the media agenda as was the case during the #MeToo and Occupy Wall Street movements (Chadwick, 2017).

Therefore, it is without doubt that non-elites are intervening in the news making process and influencing the "form and content of public discourse" through online activity and citizen journalism (Entman and Usher, 2018). This has led to more fluidity in the system of information flow which is being characterized as more "polycentric" compared to the 1960s to the 1990s, when older media logics were solely dominating (Chadwick, 2017, p. 288). Nevertheless, although the hybridity of the system is destabilizing elite power and disrupting what have become "relatively fixed patterns of interaction" between the political elite and elite traditional broadcast and print media (Chadwick, 2017, p. 286), it is not entirely diminishing the hierarchy of control over information flow. On the contrary, "elites by and large still set in motion the framing process by controlling the information they share about their preferred and actual uses of power" while institutional media continue to occupy the second level of the cascade model despite their decreased control (Entman & Usher, 2018, p. 304). Entman and

Usher's (2018) revised cascade model reflects how online platforms, algorithms and the ability to monitor and mine user activity through analytical tools build up new digital "pump-valves" that help the political elite exercise and expand their top-down power. Members of the political elite, much like any smartphone owner, constantly carry around in their pockets the tools needed to instantly and directly send their message to the public, bypassing traditional media institutions (Entman & Usher, 2018.). This is an instrument which Trump has utilized very successfully to spread his right-wing populist narrative on a large scale (Kreis, 2017). For this reason, Chadwick (2017, p. 19) argues that no understanding of power nowadays, can be complete without understanding "the relationships between social actors and technologies, because technologies enable and constrain agency" in such a "hybrid and sociotechnical" media system. Although it is not fully clear how algorithmic systems of social media platforms such as Facebook and Twitter function, leading some scholars to label them as "black boxes" (Stark & Stegmann, 2020, p. 9), it is evident that algorithms control what type of political information appears on which user's screen in line of their previously selected preferences and interests (Jürgens & Stark, 2017).

### *3.7.2 Are New Media Logics Redefying Power?*

Entman and Usher (2018, p. 301) define algorithms as the "procedures for turning input into output based on a series of calculations and ordered steps". While these calculations remain "opaque", they are utilized by social media platforms to personalize, filter and sort out users' experiences mainly based on economic incentives and the desire to maximize the time spent on the platform (Entman & Usher, 2018, p. 304). Herewith, creating so called "filter bubbles" that is "a unique universe of information for each of us" (Pariser, 2011, p. 9) as well as "echo chambers" a term used to refer to "communication situations where one is exposed only to opinions that agree with their own" (Stark & Stegmann, 2020, p. 15). It has been long known through the cognitive dissonance theory that humans prefer to associate with like-minded others while avoiding opinions that do not resonate with their own (Festinger, 1962). Algorithms feed into this desire and function in a way that reinforces "echo chambers" (see Colleoni et al., 2014). In turn, this leads to less diversity and a higher level of homophily meaning that "contact between similar people occurs at a higher rate than among dissimilar people" (McPherson et al., 2001, p. 416).

Such phenomena put society at risk of growing fragmentation and polarization that is "the ideological division of a society into different (extreme) political camps" (Stark & Stegmann, 2020, p. 150). As Moeller & Helberger (2018, p. 4) put it, "algorithmic news personalization could lead to a situation, in which the shared public sphere becomes increasingly disintegrated and breaks up into smaller issue publics." Thus, the way algorithms are built plays out in favor of ideological leaders' desire to maintain the attention of their supporters, enhance the spread of their posts and reinforce their messages (Entman & Usher, 2018; Nagel, 2019). According to Entman & Usher (2018, p. 305), those who interact with Trump's posts on social media platforms will be fed more content in the same line thereby algorithms "magnify elite power" and "enhance the efficacy of elite frames". Zhang et al. (2017) found that Twitter algorithms amplified

Trump's messages and helped increase their spread especially as they did not differentiate between attention given to his tweets due to criticism or support. Thereby, they account for making any "attempts to push back, or the slightest display of vigilant attention" on Trump's tweets work in favor of "the elevation of Trump to ever greater heights of attention" (Zhang et al., 2017, p. 3178).

Since 2014, Twitter has been pushing tweets on its users' timeline from people they don't follow based on unclear mechanisms (Dredge, 2014, October 17). As described on their official website under the "About your Twitter timeline" section:

> Additionally, when we identify a Tweet, an account to follow, or other content that's popular or relevant, we may add it to your timeline. This means you will sometimes see Tweets from accounts you don't follow. We select each Tweet using a variety of signals, including how popular it is and how people in your network are interacting with it. (Twitter, n.d.a)

According to Darcy (2019, March 22), "[i]n effect, the practice means Twitter may at times end up amplifying inflammatory political rhetoric, misinformation, conspiracy theories, and flat out lies to its users." Interestingly, the social media giant saw that this policy should be removed prior to the 2020 presidential elections as part of the platform's attempt to apply "significant product and enforcement updates that will increase context and encourage more thoughtful consideration before Tweets are amplified" (Gadde & Beykpour, 2020, October 9). Hence, Twitter announced that it will refrain from showing tweet recommendations based on popular liked content by people who are not followed by the user or even suggesting accounts "followed by" others starting October 20 "through at least the end of Election week in the US" (Gadde & Beykpour, 2020, October 9) based on the following explanation:

> These recommendations can be a helpful way for people to see relevant conversations from outside of their network, but we are removing them because we don't believe the "Like" button provides sufficient, thoughtful consideration prior to amplifying Tweets to people who don't follow the author of the Tweet, or the relevant topic that the Tweet is about. This will likely slow down how quickly Tweets from accounts and topics you don't follow can reach you, which we believe is a worthwhile sacrifice to encourage more thoughtful and explicit amplification. (Gadde & Beykpour, 2020, October 9)

Although little is yet known about the impact of the new update, a study conducted by the Statesman Data team found that Trump's original tweet growth remained unaffected by the new update with an almost steady number of retweets and an even higher number of cumulative likes, while Joe Biden's account, with almost 8 times fewer followers experienced a decrease in both types of engagement (Swindells, 2020, November 2). According to Sinan Aral, Professor of IT & Marketing Professor at MIT, the update came at the cost of smaller accounts with a limited number of followers; "The more that a Twitter policy throttles that avenue of information diffusion, the more people with a high number of direct followers are going to retain their audience than somebody with fewer followers." (Aral, 2020, November 2). Rand (2020, November 2) argues that although previous mechanisms of pushing random tweets might have amplified misinformation and partisan messages, their absence might not necessarily mean the opposite, given that the probability to be confronted with alternative viewpoints is diminished leading to higher polarization (Rand, 2020, November 2). On November 12, 2020, Twitter announced it will be reverting removing tweet recommendations given that there was no "statistically significant difference in misinformation prevalence as a result of this change" was observed (Gadde & Beykpour, 2020, November 12). Moreover, without providing real evidence Twitter asserted that the new update "prevented many people from discovering new conversations and accounts to follow." (Gadde & Beykpour, 2020, November 12.). However, if Twitter's goal is truly to open new avenues of information for its users, it is questionable why the company wants to return to more personalized tweet recommendations as it states in its latest policy:

> Our goal is to eventually replace these "liked by" and "followed by" recommendations with ones that are based on the Topics you follow or Topics we think you might like. We believe this will provide you greater control to tell us what you are and aren't interested in, which will make our recommendations more relevant to you. (Gadde & Beykpour, 2020, November 12)

In this case, if you don't engage with a certain line of content it will not pop up on your Twitter timeline even if it's popular among people you may follow. However, this does not mean that such content is not being shared anymore nor that it will not circulate on the platform anymore. On the contrary, it will only circulate among those who find it in line with their worldviews and interests which might mean even bigger "echo chambers" (Stark & Stegmann, 2020, p. 15; Swindells, 2020, November 2). If we take Eslami et al's (2015, p. 153) words into consideration on how algorithms "exert the power to shape the users' experience and even their perceptions of the world", then, what Twitter might be saying is that it will deliberately program its algorithms to limit the perception of its users towards their existing beliefs or what they indicate to the algorithms they are interested in. For example, those who follow accounts with content aligned with the political left will continue to see more in this vein. The same could be said for those interested in content that could be classified as aligned to the right of the political spectrum. This is especially alarming considering that once algorithms predict users behavior they are relatively persistent with no possibility for retraction other than complete account removal (Entman & Usher, 2018). These types of attention-based algorithms, experts say, benefited Trump by creating a "powerful ecosystem that amplifies every post" and "give an additional boost to messages based on the engagement they receive" (Dwoskin & Timberg, 2020, October 30).

### *3.7.3 From Twitter to Traditional Media*

Moreover, new technologies have established a stronger communication network between "ideological media, elites, and the public", herewith increasing and promoting the diffusion of elite frames (Entman & Usher, 2018, p. 304). Members of the political elite can now more than ever pick and choose what voices they amplify through online sharing techniques on various platforms for example by retweeting, mentions or link shares in the case of Twitter (Entman & Usher, 2018). To further emphasize their frame, self-evidently, the content chosen is mostly in line with one's own interpretations of issues and preferred policies, unless it is being shared to be undermined (Meeks, 2020). Herewith, this widens the audience reach of ideological media and reinforces its narratives (Entman & Usher, 2018). Dastgeer & Onyebadi (2020) found that Trump's retweets mainly originated from his official task force pages followed by conservative media. For example, Trump often retweets content posted by Fox News, as well as Breitbart News Network, a conservative leaning, for some also "unabashedly populist" (Wells et al., 2020) news website known for its "exceedingly favorable coverage" of Trump campaign in 2016, partisan stoking content, misleading claims and "courting Mr. Trump's most extreme followers" (Engel Bromwich, 2016, August 17; see also, Entman & Usher, 2018). Meeks (2020, p. 222) found that during Trump's nomination period prior to the 2016 elections as well as his first year in office, out of the 142 retweets originating from media outlets shared on Trump's Twitter account, 92.3% were from conservative media. Similarly, around "40% of tweets mentioned conservative media" from which roughly 83% came from "Fox, its shows, its hosts, or regular Fox commentators." (Meeks, 2020, p. 222-228). These findings also reflect how ideological media institutions by themselves also further generate and prompt leaders' initiatives (Entman & Usher, 2018). If Fox News wasn't sharing content that Trump saw as supportive of his worldview, he would have not been contributing to its spread. At the same time, Fox benefits from Trump's sharing activity thus continues to amplify his voice mainly to raise its rating and economic gains, which has led some scholars to refer to this relationship as the "Fox-Trump feedback loop" (Altheide, 2020, p. 524). Hence, the relationship between the political elite and ideological media within the hybrid systems is reciprocal and mutually strengthening "articulated by chains of dependence and interdependence" (Chadwick, 2017, p. 19).

Indeed, Trump succeeded in utilizing social media platforms to bypass traditional media institutions by flooding online public forums with unfiltered messages sent directly from the President. Sometimes this was even carried out unilaterally to the surprise of his own staff members and White House officials, leaving journalists who, under older media logics acquired news first, chasing to catch up to content that would arrive to the screens of millions before being subjected to journalistic reflection or fact checking (Chadwick, 2017; Entman & Usher, 2018). As a result, in many cases professional media coverage even on social media came as a reaction to Trump's use of new media logics (Chadwick, 2017). In fact, only around one third of voters who have seen Trump Tweets spotted them directly on Twitter; the rest were exposed to them through mainstream media (Altheide, 2020). Therefore, as Wells et al. (2020) argue, Trump not only bypassed professional media, he systematically succeeded in attracting their attention and influencing their coverage regardless of where outlets stood on the political spectrum whether from the far-right as Breitbart or more left leaning outlets like Mother Jones and the New Yorker. In their study, Wells et al. (2020) applied two statistical methods; Granger causality and autoregression on a large-scale longitudinal data set from 25 US media outlets to examine the relationship between Trump's Twitter activity, campaign events as well as poll numbers and attention given to him by professional media outlets defined as at least two mentions within one article. They found a consistent causal relationship between the number of retweets on @realDonaldTrump and the amount of attention he received from professional media outlets. Meaning that the higher the number of retweets the higher his mentions in media coverage while public events did not cause such a consistent effect (Wells et al., 2020).

More interestingly, it seems like Trump was fully aware of this dynamic as it was proven that he tended to tweet more when the amount of attention given to him by professional media was decreasing (Wells et al., 2020). This adds weight to Chadwick's (2017, p. 262) argument that Trump continuously used Twitter "to stoke the fires of coverage" and reflects Schroeder's (2018, p. 62) description of the role of Twitter as "a transmission belt to visibility in traditional media". Trump said it himself in an interview with ABC News' Journalist George Stephanopoulos in June 2019: "I put it out, and then it goes onto your platform. It goes onto ABC. It goes onto the networks. It goes onto all over the cable. It's an incredible way of communicating." (Trump, 2019, June 17). Wells et al. (2020, p. 676) assert that their findings reflect "both the hybrid nature of the media environment and the significance of social media as an engine with the potential to push attention to populists into every corner of the mediasphere". To better understand President Trump's communication style including his populist leaning rhetoric the next chapter will provide an overview of his preferred use of language.

# 4 Literature Review

## 4.1 Trump's Communication Style

### *4.1.1 Populism*

From day one, Trump's adopted rhetoric echoed populist beliefs including anti-immigrant and nationalist sentiment (Rice-Oxley & Kaila, 2018, December 3). "For too long, a small group in our nation's capital has reaped the rewards of government while the people have borne the cost.", he said in his 2017 inauguration speech (Trump, 2017, January 20). This fits directly into Mudde & Rovira Kaltwasser's (2017, p. 6) definition of populism as a:

> thin-centred ideology that considers society to be ultimately separated into two homogeneous and antagonistic camps, "the pure people" versus the "corrupt elite," and which argues that politics should be an expression of the volonté générale (general will) of the people.

For Taggart (200, p. 1) populist leaders are "most extraordinary individuals [leading] the most ordinary of people". According to Müller (2016, p. 101) what makes them extraordinary is not only that they are "antielitists" but also "antipluralist" as populist leaders advocate that they "represent the people" or more accurately "the 100 percent" of the people. But this can never be realistic nor applicable as the term, the people, in itself may only come in plural (Habermas, as cited in Müller, 2016). However, such a logic enables populists to dismiss arguments as immoral and frame political rivals as “enemies of the people” in need to be excluded, including governmental bodies and their respective apparatuses (Müller, 2016, p. 3). This puts the upholding of the system of checks and balances within a political system like the one in the US under continuous threat (Kyle & Meyer, 2020). As a result, populists refuse to accept any oppositional argument as legitimate, turning political debates into a question of right and wrong in which their answer is always the “morally pure” one and the others the “morally inferior” (Müller, 2016, p. 20). As Müller (2016, p. 3) puts it, populist leaders, “thrive on conflict and encourage polarization” using morality as an argument. In that way, and since only they speak the voice of the people, populist presidents behave as if they can “issue something like an imperative mandate that tells politicians exactly what they have to do in government” thereby representing a picture that there is actually “no need for the endless political debates nor the “messy back-and-forth of deliberating in Congress or other national assemblies” (Müller, 2016, p. 30). This all makes populism a threat to democracy, especially the inability to recognize societal diversity as an undeniable fact and a fundamental necessity for the success of any nation in which all people are free and equal. Thus, when a populist leader governs they reflect three main features:

(1) attempts to hijack the state apparatus

(2) corruption and “mass clientelism” (trading material benefits or bureaucratic favors for political support by citizens who become the populists’ “clients”)

(3) efforts systematically to suppress civil society (Müller, 2016, p. 4)

### *4.1.2 A Man in the Street Communication Style*

Populism is not only an ideology but also a communication style that has been appearing in US political context since the 1830s with its most recent resurgence being documented since the start of Trump's election campaign in 2016 (Bucy et al. 2020; de Vreese et al., 2018). It can be perceived as "an act of speech" (Block, & Negrine, 2017, p. 179) and a "mode of presentation" (Engesser, 2017, p. 1280) that employs language, signs or visual elements to connect with a subset of the population - viewed as the 100 percent of the people by the leaders thus the only legitimate source of political authority - while demonizing the others (Block, & Negrine, 2017, p. 179). Kyle and Meyer (2020) classify Trump as a cultural populist which is the populist variation associated with right-wing nationalist politics. Jair Bolsonaro, the President of Brazil, Benjamin Netanyahu, the Prime Minister of Israel and Narendra Modi, the Prime Minister of India are also considered cultural populists. The main definition of social conflict for cultural populists' rests upon the idea that there is only one homogeneous group that defines the native-members of the nation, while, the other such as immigrants, criminals and religious minorities are perceived as outsiders (Kyle & Meyer, 2020). "Cultural populists tend to emphasize religious traditionalism, law and order, anti-immigration positions, and national sovereignty." (Kyle & Meyer, 2020, p. 7). Socio-economic populism on the other hand, incorporates left-wing leaders who frame the big business and capital owners as the outsider who unjustly benefit from the working class causing them economic and social disadvantages. In that sense, former Venezuelan President Hugo Chávez and US politician Bernie Sanders are perceived as socio-economic populists (Kyle & Meyer, 2020, p. 7).

Trump's communication style is in line with that of a cultural populism, known for its simple choice of words and sentence structures (Bos et al., 2011). It favors simplification and straightforwardness over complexity with the goal of appearing as an ordinary member of the public (Bos et al., 2011). A "man in the street communication styles" as Albertazzi and McDonnell (2008, p. 2) put it, directly feeding into populist core desire to build an image of us vs. them by positioning oneself on the side of the public and outside the main political elite group (Müller, 2016). Simplification also includes reducing problems to single causes and treatments that rotate around the necessity of having one's strong leadership and the ability to take fast measures (Bos et al., 2011; Bucy et al., 2020). In that way, "the whole world is depicted in black and white without any shades of gray (Engesser, 2017, p. 1285). Populists and Trump alike, systematically employ "dramatisation" which is the "need to generate tension in order to build up support [...] by denouncing the tragedies that would befall the community if it were to be deprived of its defences" (Albertazzi, 2007 p. 335). To achieve this, words that reflect emotions are favored over objectivity and neutrality as these are more useful in evoking "fear, and anger, toward perceived adversaries while projecting hope onto the populist leader who promises to deliver the masses from their plight" (Bucy et al., 2020, p. 637). Consider, for example, Trump's use of the words: bad, sad, boring or terrible to describe political issues or actions of his democratic opponents (Hages, 2017). Emotionalizing language thus also incorporates conveying negative feelings towards the political opponents who are presented standing in the way of a better future for the nation (Bucy et al., 2020). After conducting a content analysis of campaign speeches by all candidates, Oliver & Rahn (2016) concluded that the 2016 elections brought with it a general rise in populist rhetoric in the US. However, Trump stood out as the "populist par excellence" as his speeches were mainly directed towards targeting political elites with the help of simple and repetitive language that envoys blame and evokes "foreign threats and collective notions of 'our' and 'they'" (Oliver & Rahn, 2016, p. 193).

### *4.1.3 Direct Causation*

According to Lakoff (2016, July 23), Trump managed to win the 2016 Republican presidential primaries because he was able to speak to people's anger offering solutions in terms of direct causation rather than systematic causation which requires more complex understanding of how problems come to stand through "chains of direct causes, interacting causes, feedback loops, and probabilistic causes". Direct causation, on the other hand, is more simplified and can be easily explained in clear language and grammar. For example, following Trump's logic, the number of immigrants is rising? No problem, we will build a wall. The US is experiencing increased mass shootings? The answer is simple; equip more people with guns to be able to shoot the shooter. Low priced foreign goods are replacing locally produced goods? Raise tariffs on them. Some terrorists kill in the name of Islam? Ban all Muslims (Lakoff, 2016, July 23). These types of solutions resonate because they don't require putting effort into tracking all the possible combined societal, political or economic causes behind what some see as problems. It also calls out a single person or something to blame and indicates higher possibilities of seeing quick change rather than a long process with no exact time limit. For example, adding the word Islamic before terrorism suggest one name as an enemy: Muslims. "This is the basis for the Trumpian metaphor that Naming is Identifying" (Lakoff 2016, July 23).

### *4.1.4 Political Incorrectness*

Trump speaks "force, aggression, anger, and no shame" while intentionally distancing himself away from political correctness to capture the attention of those who feel like it restricts their freedom of speech (Lakoff, 2016, July 23). The term political correctness has been on the rise in US political and cultural debates since the 1980s (Schafer, 2017). It describes adapting a language and argumentative line that gives "excessive attention to the sensibilities of those who are seen as different from the norm (women, gays and lesbians, Black people, the disabled)" (Mills 2003, p. 89). Barack Obama, for example, is known for his mastering of politically correct language (Theye & Melling, 2018). Trump, on the other hand, openly states that he has no interest in being politically correct as it just takes "too much time" and "too much effort" (Trump for President, 2016). Instead, there are so many things that should be done but can never be "if we just stay politically correct" (Trump for President, 2016). According to Schafer (2017, p. 8) Trump adapts and advertises a narrative that portrays political incorrectness as a manner of truth telling which in fact "normalizes backstage racist framing of issues". Such frames get reinforced by Trump's use of repetition as an integral part of his communication as well as his consistent employment of the same catchphrases like "Believe Me" or "Many people are saying" which as explained in the theory section further elevates the power of his frames (Entman, 2003; Lakoff, 2017).

### *4.1.5 Hyperbole*

Hyperbole as a language tool is also continuously spotted in Trump's speeches (Abbas, 2019; Kayam, 2018; Mendoza-Denton, 2020). It is "a regular feature of informal talk that speakers exaggerate narrative, descriptive and argumentative features and make assertions that are overstated, literally impossible, inconceivable or counterfactual" (McCarthy & Carter, 2003, p. 149). Exaggeration can be used in opposite directions for example to make something appear smaller or bigger, better or worse, beneficial or harmful. For this reason, Christodoulidou (2011) describes hyperbole as a way of structuring a reality in which there are two competing realities which explains why populists systematically employ hyperbole; it makes it easier to draw the black and white picture with no gray as mentioned by Engesser (2017). In classical rhetoric, exaggerated amplification or enlargement is referred to as meiosis while auxesis describes the opposite; attenuation and reduction (Smith 1657; Al-Azzawi & Hameed, 2020). Hyperbole is carried out in various forms including adjectives or adverbs that exaggerate size, degree or intensity such as Trump's all-time favorites: tremendous, enormous, massive, greatest or very much, alot etc. (Kayam, 2018; McCarthy & Carter, 2003). Over statements of time, numbers and quantity such as tons, millions of, masses, and a billion years (McCarthy & Carter, 2003). Sometimes hyperbole comes as mere impossible expressions like telling someone "I'm in a coma" while actually standing in front of them (Christodoulidou, 2011). In politics hyperbole is used for "emphasising the seriousness of the situation, the urgency of action, criticising the political opponent and praising one's own party or policies" (Claridge, 2011, p. 265). Politicians mainly employ it to draw a positive image of oneself and a negative one of the opponents (Dijik, 2006). Hence, it is also a strong method of manipulation and persuasion to gain interest and marshal support (Van Dijk, 2006) as Trump himself said it to the ghost writer of his book *The Art of the Deal*:

> I play to people's fantasies. People may not always think big themselves, but they can still get very excited by those who do. That's why a little hyperbole never hurts. People want to believe that something is the biggest and the greatest and the most spectacular. I call it truthful hyperbole. It's an innocent form of exaggeration—and a very effective form of promotion. (Trump & Schwartz, 1987, p. 58)

#### *4.1.6 Insult Politics and Mocking Rhetoric*

Trump is also known for performing insult politics and mocking rhetoric (Winberg, 2017). Insults go beyond criticizing the opponent or casting them in negative terms as they carry offensive and degrading meanings (Clocker, 2020; Wellsby 2010). For Winbery (2017, p. 3) insults refer to "ad hominem attacks of a disparaging nature aimed at an individual or group." (Winbery, 2017, p. 3). For example, in 2018, Trump described Haiti and El Salvador as "shithole" countries (Dawsey, 2018, January 12). He also publicly used words like “fat pig”, “horseface” and “dogs” to refer to women (Walsh, 2018, October 17). It is also common for Trump to turn his insults into some sort of nicknames for his opponents “low-energy Jeb” (Jeb Bush), “Crooked Hillary” (Hillary Clinton), “Crazy Bernie” (Bernie Sanders) and “Sleepy Joe” (Judd, 2020, March 2; Ross & Rivers, 2020). Since nicknames are rooted in comedy as “a play upon form: that is, as a joke, or rather, the punchline of a joke” they serve as entertainment methods even when employed in politics (Blok, 2001, p.157). In this way, they help capture attention and provide supporters with means of further isolating the opponents. As Hall et al. (2016, p. 86) explain: “By mocking the subject and making the named person look foolish, nicknames give special powers to the provider.” Nearly two weeks before the 2020 election day, Trump described Anthony Fauci, the director of the National Institute of Allergy and Infectious Diseases as an “idiot” and a “disaster” who has been around for “500 years” in combination of both hyperbole and insults (Collinson, 2020, October 20). Mocking and insulting a member of the White House Coronavirus Task Force during a period of rising COVID-19 infection numbers in the country reflects Colcker’s (2020, p. 6) argument that Trump does not use insults to attack but also to “deflect attention away from important issues” and “undermine the attainment of progressive policies”. It also indicates that little has changed in Trump’s communication style during the pandemic. On the contrary, his attacking language has been furthered to include science, scientists and governmental health institutions, leaving the country in a more vulnerable position (Hetherington & Ladd, 2020, May 1). Thus, the next chapter aims to provide an overview of what research has established so far about Trump's framing patterns during the COVID-19 pandemic also in comparison to other world leaders.

## 4.2 Framing The COVID-19 Pandemic

Historically, the media and the political elite predominantly relied on war and conflict frames when discussing diseases such as AIDS, tuberculosis and cancer (Sontag 1978; 1989; Annas, 1995; Montgomery, 1991; Worboys, 2000). Former US President Richard Nixon's activation of the "war on cancer frame" in the 1970s is a particular example of this (Wallis & Nerlich, 2005). War frames are usually constructed through the use of militaristic terminology such as "fighting," "battling," or "combating" the "enemy" which, in return, results in the classifications of those affected by the disease as either "victims" or "survivors" (Grant & Hundley, 2009, p. 16). Even when the media was able to distance its language away from war and military metaphors as was the case in British newspapers coverage of SARS in 2003, they still failed to use alternative non-violent or scientific language and in turn stimulated an image of SARS as a "killer" (Wallis and Nerlich, 2005). Similarly, studies about the framing of the COVID-19 pandemic show that neither the media nor various members of the political elite were able to abandon the war frame (Benziman, 2020; Islentyeva, 2020; Sondermann & Ulbert, 2020). French President Emmanuel Macron said it to his nation loud and clear in his speech on March 16, 2020: "We are at war" (Macron, 2020, March 16). British Prime Minister Borris Johnson (2020, March 23) similarly asserted: "But in this fight we can be in no doubt that each and every one of us is directly enlisted. Each and every one of us is now obliged to join together." While US President Trump declared himself a "wartime President" that is "battling an invisible enemy" (Trump, 2020, March 23a).

Leaders resort to defining health crises as wars not only because it allows them to contextualize circumstances within a framework that the public is familiar with - an existing schemata of interpretation that requires less cognitive effort - but also because it allows them to issue measures based on wartime rules. Thus, giving themselves "more leverage in how they ask the public to act and what they ask the public to accept." (Benziman, 2020, p. 253). During war and conflict, all circumstances change, people are expected to "rally around the flag", overcome internal disputes in order to fight the common enemy, be more patriotic including making personal sacrifices for the benefit of the country and success of the nation as well as "learn to accept the idea that there will be casualties and victims" (Benziman, 2020, p. 248; see also, Ariely, 2016; Bar-Tal, 2013; Bar Tal & Staub, 1997; Hetherington & Nelson, 2003; Milla, Putra, & Umam, 2019; Mueller, 1970; Somerville, 1981). At the same time, casting circumstances in terms of war, allows leaders to suggest having a plan or a concrete "strategy" on how to "win" and "defeat" the enemy, thereby reflecting the notion that there will be an end to the suffering at one point, if the public follows and cooperates (Benziman, 2020, p. 254). Indeed, previous studies indicate that the public is more willing to comply with governmental measures when the country experiences a security threat (LaFree & Adamczyk, 2017).

In his inductive qualitative content analysis of Trump and Johnson's speeches, press conferences and statement releases from March 2020, Benziman (2020) found that both leaders employed similar language and lines of argumentation, with slight differences due to Johnson's infection. Both mainly framed the COVID-19 pandemic as a "war" by referring to the virus as an "invisible killer" and "hidden enemy" (Benziman, 2020, p. 53). Although Trump and Johnson indicated that the situation will not be easy and that worse times are yet to come, perhaps even with more loss of lives, they incited hope by suggesting that the enemy is "beatable" and "victory is possible". Two types of plans were presented to the public to achieve this goal; The economic plan which entailed either reassurance that the respective countries will not run out of food and consumer goods in the present (March 2020), or promises to help recover the economy in the future. The first type of economic response found by Benziman (2020) could be seen as a reaction to the rise of panic buying documented in March 2020 in countries all over the world, including in the US and UK (IRI, 2020, April 23). Panic buying refers to "building up inventories in excess of current consumption needs" (Keane & Neal, 2021, p. 86). For example, spendings on paper goods including toilet paper rose by 217% in the US and 134% in the UK between 9 and 15 March, 2020 compared to the year 2019 (IRI, 2020, April 23). The health plan was divided into instructions on how to slow the spread of the virus and information about governmental measures being taken. However, while the leaders took responsibility for finding economic solutions, they mainly framed the public as the responsible agent for carrying out the health plan. Complying with state proposed changing measures such as social distancing was defined as "national- collective action of patriotism" and "the new version of unity" thus worth the "sacrifice" of one's own desires (Benziman, 2020, p. 251). Medical teams were framed as the "heros" and the "most patriotic figures in this war" (Benziman, 2020, p. 251). Benziman (2020) argues that although both leaders defined the pandemic as a global problem or more accurately, a war the whole world is fighting, each of them drew a picture that his own country is doing better than others. The reason for this, according to each leader, is not because of the collective effort of the nation, although they continuously appealed to that, but because he himself is the leader of the nation who is doing a great job. Both Trump and Johnson practiced positive self-rating, according to the author. This was done through comparing one's action and country to other countries, quoting other leaders and experts "saying they did a great job" and more subtly through sending condolences to other countries' leaders "thereby highlighting the better situation in their country" (Benziman, 2020, p. 252). Benziman's findings correspond with Sondermann and Ulbert's (2020, p. 315) argument that, although the COVID-19 pandemic is a global health crisis "it has been met in national understandings and corresponding national responses. These were mostly exclusively focused on protecting their own citizens or framed as enhancing national interests." Nevertheless, since Benziman's (2020) study focused on war framing it fails to offer an interpretation of Trump's use of the term Chinese virus. It does, however, reflect the binary picture war frames build about reality, one in which there is either winning or losing with no gray area in between. Despite the fact that gray areas speak more for the COVID-19 pandemic situations and it's "new kind of reality where the routine of life is neither a "'war' nor the ordinary life" as argued by Benziman (2020, p. 254). Moreover, the danger of thinking in war frames is that "it creates images of 'us' vs. 'it' as a unified 'we' against an outside, suddenly emerging threat." (Sondermann & Ulbert, 2020, p. 311). In that sense, Sondermann and Ulbert (2020, p. 314) argue that

Trump's naming of the coronavirus as the Chinese Virus or Wuhan Virus presents the COVID-19 pandemic as a "traditional security issue" and China as "a source of that threat". It focuses on deflecting blame by portraying the health crisis as something "unforeseeable" and "not our fault". Thereby, "shortening complex lines of causality and responsibility and privileging national answers." (Sondermann & Ulbert, 2020, p. 315). This line of reasoning reflects Trump's favoring of direct causation over systemic causation explained in the previous section. Also, since security threats normally bring with them danger and fear, using simple causation of a foreign threat allows leaders to propose "reactive emergency measures" rather than "long-term systemic approaches" and "transmits a sense of control" thereby shifting power to the executive and creating a cycle of securitizing the COVID-19 pandemic (Sondermann & Ulbert, 2020, p. 315). It was also part of his long-known reliance on the politics of fear such as fear from immigrants and fear from Muslims (Keller, 2016; Altheide, 2020). Thus, he tried to use the pandemic to reinforce his border and security politics. "Trump often referred to borders and walls to play to Americans' fears and to protect them from immigrants" (Altheide, p. 529). However, while magnifying fear from the "others", Altheide (2020, p. 521) finds that between December 2019 and May 2020, Trump mainly downplayed the seriousness of the COVID-19 pandemic and defined the coronavirus as "benign and insignificant" in his official as well as Twitter communication content. He continuously told the public that "there is nothing to worry about" and failed to give advice on how to slow the spread of the coronavirus (Altheide, 2020, p. 521). One of Trump's main tactics of downplaying the pandemic was through comparing it to the seasonal flu (Hatcher, 2020). He even constructed an image of prevention measures such as social distancing and lockdown as attacks on his program and agenda. For him they were just "bad for business" as Altheide (2020, 534) puts it. "One tragic consequence is that the US is and will remain the epicentre of the pandemic accounting for >20% of global cases and deaths with <5% of the population" (Alter, 2020, p. 2).

At the same time, Trump showed more concern about the economy than the public health and tried to frame the pandemic as a "a hoax that the Democrats were promoting to hinder President Trump's reelection bid" (Altheide, 2020, p. 522) as well as an overhyped and exaggerated "media hoax" (Borah, 2020, p. 2). To further reinforce his dismissive narrative, Trump continued to practice his known naming and attacking politics by referring to media outlets as "Fake News CNN", "LameStream media" and "Fake News NYT" (Borah, 2020, p. 3). Similarly, Meyer (2020) found that Trump and the Brazilian President Bolsonaro, who the author identifies as cultural populists, mainly downplayed the COVID-19 pandemic and can be characterized as being anti-science. For them, the pandemic represented an "opportunity to draw cultural dividing lines with opponents to strengthen their own positions." (Meyer, 2020, p. 3). Crayne and Medeiros (2020) similarly argue that Bolsonaro's handling of the COVID-19 pandemic was mainly negative, dismissive and prioritizing of economic actions over public health actions. His narrative mirrored Trump's "blame politics" towards the media (Altheide, 2020, p. 529), by accusing them of exaggerating the pandemic situation resulting in an unnecessary "hysteria" (Bolsonaro, 2020, March 23). Studies show a high resemblance degree between Trump and Bolserano's sense-making of the COVID-19 Pandemic (Junk & Peez, 2020, November 3; Mannion & Speed, 2020; Meyer, 2020; Sánchez et al., 2021).

Columnist Max Boot offers a combat summary of the two in The Washington Post:

> Bolsonaro is like a cartoon version of the U.S. president, who is already a cartoon version of a demagogue. Like Trump, Bolsonaro has dismissed the threat (he called the virus a "measly cold"). Like Trump, Bolsonaro has feuded with governors and health officials who want to order a lockdown; he even fired his health minister for urging strict social isolation. Like Trump, Bolsonaro has failed to do enough testing and touts hydroxychloroquine as a miracle cure. Like Trump, Bolsonaro fails to display empathy: Asked about Brazil's death count overtaking China's, Bolsonaro said last week, "So what? I'm sorry. What do you expect me to do?" And like Trump, Bolsonaro has urged people to go back to work, saying, "Sometimes, the cure is worse than the disease." (Boot, 2020, May 6)

Islentyeva's (2020) findings come in congruence with Benziman (2020), however the author notes that Trump's reliance on the war metaphor was stronger than Johnson's. In her qualitative discourse analysis of the political framing of the pandemic, Islentyeva (2020) further included Russian President Vladimir Putin and German Chancellor Angela Merkel. Five speeches delivered by each leader between the beginning of March and June 2020 formed the corpus of the pilot study. According to the author, Merkel and Putin were able to distance themselves from framing the pandemic as a war, with limited exceptions such as descriptions of medical and social care workers as "heroes" and "frontline protectors". Instead, Merkel mainly framed the pandemic as a "challenge", "dynamic situation" and a "difficult ordeal", the government response to it as a "task" while appealing to the public to "unite together" to help accomplish it (Islentyeva, 2020, p. 169). She was the only leader to try and personalize the pandemic by emphasizing that infected people are not just numbers but "fathers and mothers, grandfathers and grandmothers, and partners" (Islentyeva, 2020, p. 169). Crayne and Medeiros (2020, p. 7) argue that Merkel's sense making of the COVID-19 pandemic mirrors "text-book pragmatic response" as her definition of the pandemic in speeches and interviews is always problem-focused with few appeals to the emotions of the German public but rather to their rationale. Thus, she relies heavily on scientific evidence in her line of reasoning avoiding sensational arguments and overrating positive developments (Crayne & Medeiros, 2020). Unlike Trump who, according to Altheide (2020), was against science and did integrate it in his communication. Oltermann (2020, April 26) argues that even Merkel's critics "have come to appreciate a politician who is on safer ground explaining the importance of decimal places than projecting great visions of the future."

Putin framed the pandemic in a more general and tranquil manner; a "situation" that is "difficult or "not easy" (Islentyeva, 2020, p. 172). He portrayed governmental measures as "tactics" or a "strategy" and the spread of the virus as a "threat" (Islentyeva, 2020, p. 171). However, unlike Benziman (2020), Islentyeva (2020) does not directly link these words to war framing patterns by arguing that they are "semantically broad" and "imply a planned set of coherent actions for achieving something" (Islentyeva, 2020, p.

172). Both Putin and Merkel gave a positive turn to the word fight by connecting it to peace, argues Islentyeva (2020). Merkel discussed fighting to bring back peace and prosperity to Europe while Putin mentioned struggling for peace. However, the main difference between the two is that Merkel did not want to show that her country is standing in isolation of other countries, while Putin, similar to Johnson and Trump (Benziman, 2020), aimed at highlighting the uniqueness of his country's handling of the virus. Nonetheless, Putin made no contrasts to other countries but rather focused on the specialty of the ancestors of the Russian nation (Islentyeva, 2020). In a way, Putin's rhetoric "echoes Trump's Idea of (US) exceptionalism" (Islentyeva, 2020, 176). Islentyeva (2020) study also provides more recent proof that hyperbole remained an integral part of Trump's communication style as he used words like "big, tremendous, fantastic, a lot, and total" to draw a picture of the US as the "the only powerful country in the world" (Islentyeva, 2020, 167). Merkel on the other hand, unlike all three leaders, employed contrasts to other countries in a more positive manner by inviting the public and her government to learn from the success stories of other countries such as South Korea (Crayne & Medeiros, 2020).

In his attempt to move away from research centrism on Europe and North America, Rajandan (2020) conducted a qualitative content analysis of interviews, speeches and statements given by Yassin Muhyiddin the Prime Minister of Malaysia and Lee Hsien Loong the Prime Minister of Singapore between March and May 2020. Focusing only on identifying metaphors, Ranjandan's (2020) findings go in line with Benziman's (2020) and Islentyeva (2020). Both South Asian leaders also relied on war metaphors to discuss the COVID-19 pandemic with very limited scientific descriptions of the virus. For example, Muhyiddin referred to the coronavirus as the "silent enemy" while Lee called it a "common enemy" (Rajandan, 2020, p 264). Similar to the French President, Muhyiddin told his nation on March 27, 2020: "We are a nation at war" (Rajandan, 2020, p. 264). Lee, in line with Johnson and Trump, warned the public that the "battle" will be long and requires sacrifices especially from the medical staff who were referred to as front liners (Rajandan, 2020, 256; Benziman, 2020). However, he framed the coronavirus as a "hit" on the economy, which the author argues "makes the Singaporean economy a casualty" (Ragandan, 2020, p. 264).

Two points stand out in Rajandan's (2020) results. First, both leaders' frequent usage of inclusive collective pronouns such (we, our, and us) when addressing the public. "Their use inspires shared reactions, making it virtuous to adhere to these directives" according to Ragandan (2020, p. 264). Halliday and Hasan (1976, p. 53) argue that politicians use the pronoun we, to signify the "particular group of individuals with which the speaker wishes to identify". Previous research shows that when politicians employ collective pronouns they are more likely to receive favorable reactions (van Dick et al., 2007) or be viewed as charismatic (Platow et al., 2006). Steffens and Haslam (2013, p. 1) concluded that victorious Prime Ministerial candidates in Australia, made 61% more references to collective pronouns in their pre-election speeches than those who lost, indicating that "electoral endorsement is associated with leaders' capacity to engage with, and speak on behalf of, a collective identity". In his inauguration speech from 2017, Trump used the collective pronouns "we" 49 times compared to 3 times uses of "I" and 9 times “you” (Wahyuningsih, 2018). Based on a qualitative analysis the author concluded that that “we” was employed to “embrace the American people as a part of his position” and represent an existing relationship between him, his family and the American People (Wahyuningsih, 2018, p. 348). Second, Rajandan (2020) pointed out Muhyiddin’s framing of the “fighting” against the coronavirus as a religious responsibility. He said, “we are fighting a jihad against COVID-19” as translated in Rajandan (2020, p. 265). Jihad is an Arabic term mentioned in the Quran which means according to the Council on American-Islamic Relations the “individual struggle for spiritual self perfection” and is used by Muslims to signify “rightful strife, endeavor or struggle to repel evil. Such struggle can be of intellectual, mental, physical or material nature and is done only to win the pleasure of God” (CAIR, n.d). Since Islam is the official religion of Malaysia with the highest number of followers in the country compared to other religions (Nordin, 2018), Rajandan’s (2020) findings show how a war frame can be transferred to fit into different cultural context but with the same goal as mentioned by Benziman (2020): evoke the willingness to sacrifice. As previously mentioned, a frame that fits into the common culture of the recipients becomes more “noticeable, understandable, memorable and emotionally charged” (Entman, 2003, p. 417). Paulus (2020, May 22) argues that it is precisely because of this same reason that the German Chancellor avoided using the war frame; War frames simply do not resonate within the German culture because of its bitter history during World War II.

After qualitatively analyzing 203 viral tweets (+500 likes) posted by world leaders of G7 countries between mid-November, 2020 and mid-March 2020 about the

COVID-19 pandemic (Canada, France, Italy, Japan, UK, US) as well as President of the EU Council and President of the EU Commission (Germany was excluded because the German Chancellor does not have a personal Twitter account), Rufai and Bunce (2020, p. 511) concluded that the majority of the tweets were dominated by an "informative theme" defined as "seeking to share information or updates" while 9.4% were "seeking to boost morale or galvanize" and 6.9% were "seeking to raise a point of political debate". Interestingly, all of the tweets labeled as political (6.9%) originated from Trump's Twitter account. These findings reflect a high degree of politicization of the pandemic practiced by Trump in comparison to leaders of other major world countries. Several US senators argued in a call for investigation addressed to the US Pandemic Response Accountability Committee (PRAC) that, "[p]resident Trump and his advisors have repeatedly put their partisan political interests ahead of the health and welfare of the American people." (Warren et al., 2020, p. 1). Drylie-Carey et al. (2020) findings come in consonance with Rufai and Bunce (2020), who found that European leaders (UK, Italy, France, Spain) as well as the World Health Organisation (WHO) representative Tedros Adhanom and Ursula Von der Leyen President of the European Union (EU), mainly used their Twitter account as a "medium for information" between mid-March and mid-April. However, the authors criticize the leaders for falling to reflect an image of themselves following the counter measures they were asking the public to comply with, as they frequently appeared without wearing masks or practicing social distancing. No similar studies were found about Trump's Twitter content. However, in his sentiment analysis of Trump's twitter messages between mid-November and mid-March, 2020, Yaqub (2020) found a negative correlation between sentiments of his messages and the number of infections in the US. Thus, indicating that with the rise of infections, Trump started shifting his tone towards a more negative one given that his messages were mainly positive in January and February.

# 5 Methodology

## 5.1 Context and Time Period

The first clusters of infections with novel coronavirus (SARS-CoV-2) were reported in Wuhan, China on December 31, 2019, while the case outside China was first registered in Thailand two weeks later (Reuters, 2020a, September 29). Shortly after, the US reported its earliest detection of the virus on January 21 (CDC, 2020, January 21). However, Trump didn't publish any tweet related to the virus until three days later. Considering that the time period of any study "forms the parameters for defining the universe from which a sample is to be drawn (Linström & Marais, 2012, p. 29), the time period of this study was set between January 24, 2020 and January 8, 2021. The duration was chosen to be that long in order to provide a comprehensive overview of Trump's entire tweeting activity in relation to the pandemic and highlight possible changes over time in his elite frames as the highest ranking official of the US government.

To help achieve this goal, the study period was broken down into four different time periods; epidemic period, pandemic period, pre-election period and post-election period. The goal is to enable the contextualization of tweets based on their time of publishing. Pan and Kosicki (1993, p. 57), argue that using framing as a methodological strategy requires "constructing and processing discourse or characteristics of the discourse itself". To place tweets within their exact context a chronological timeline of pandemic related main events was developed and can be found in appendix A. This becomes more evident considering that this paper is based on a qualitative content analysis approach thus providing context for the study brings a systematic perspective on the issue and helps explain the meaning of text in relation to the outer circumstances that surrounded it (Linström & Marais, 2012).

The first time period includes the early outbreak stages of the disease up until the WHO characterized the outbreak as a pandemic on March 11, 2020 (Tedros Adhanom, 2020, March 11). According to the CDCs' official website (2012, May 18), an epidemic refers to "an increase, often sudden, in the number of cases of a disease above what is normally expected in that population in that area" while the word pandemic driven from the Greek words "pan" (all) and "demos" (people) is used to describe a disease widespread on international level (Wan, 2020, March 11). The CDC defines a pandemic as "an epidemic that has spread over several countries or continents, usually affecting a large number of people" (CDC, 2012, May 18). In that way, a start of pandemic marks the start of a more advanced stage of an epidemic which resulted in the distinction between the first two periods. However, not necessary in the sense that the virus has become deadlier but that the widespread of the disease is no more bound to a limited geographical area and is thereby harder to control and in more require of international concern as it puts the entire world population in question (Wan, 2020, March 11). According to WHO Director-General Dr. Tedros, the naming of the pandemic came as the organizations' last recourse to "ring the alarm bell loud and clear" (Tedros, 2020, March 11). In his speech declaring the naming of COVID-19 as a pandemic he said: "There's been so much attention on one word" calling for the need to give much more attention to words that are of higher importance and in need for wider action and change;

"Prevention, Preparedness, Public health and Political leadership" (Tedros, 2020, March 11). In that manner the question here is: What were the main messages behind Trumps' political leadership on Twitter as the world population, including Americans, are learning to live in a pandemic?

On September 29, 2020 the first presidential debate between Donald Trump and Joe Biden took place, marking the first time the two candidates met face to face for a political debate since the beginning of the outbreak. During the debate, Trump bragged about not wearing a mask in public and tried to use this precautionary measure as a way to mock his opponent Joe Biden for wearing "the biggest mask I've seen" (USA Today, 2020). Three days later, he announced his infection with the disease along with first lady Melania in a tweet which became the most retweeted one in Trump's History (TweetBinder, 2020). Hence, major events related to the President's handling of the coronavirus happened throughout this week which called for the creation of the third time period in order to be able to look at; if and how Trump's infection with the disease, as well as the ultimate nearing of the elections, affected his language framing patterns of the pandemic. This leads us to the question; What aspects of the pandemic did Trump tweets try to shift the focus on?

The fourth time period starts with the end of election day on November 4, 2020. Nothing Trump says at this point may actually affect the number of votes he gets. The question here remains: How does Trump's framing patterns after votes have been cast relate to his framing patterns in previous periods? Meanwhile, the US became the first country in the world to surpass 10 million cases, on November 9 (see appendix).

However, on December 11, 2020 the US Food and Drug Administration (FDA) issued its first Emergency Use Authorization (EUA) to the COVID-19 vaccine developed by Pfizer and BioNTech marking the beginning of a new era of the COVID-19 pandemic in the US in which vaccination can start (see appendix).

## 5.2 Sampling

To collect relevant tweets posted on @realDonalndTrump, the official Twitter account of the 45th president of the United States within the defined time period, a search was performed on the trump archiver website (www.thetrumparchive.com) with the help of the following filtering keywords: COVID19 | coronavirus | corona | covid | Covid-19 | Virus | chinavirus | "chinese virus" | pandemic | vaccine | masks | CDC | "World Health Organization" | W.H.O | FDA | Fauci | NIH |"social distancing" | quarantine | "Stay home" | lockdown | Hydroxychloroquine | Covid19pandemic | coronavirusoutbreak | Outbreak | Plague.

The trump archiver website developed in 2016 operates by a Search/REST API and uses an API tool called Tweepy to check Trump's tweets every 60 seconds and archive them into one database (Trump archiver, n.d). It enables filtering tweets based on the publication date and device type, it was posted from as well as the occurrence of one or more keywords within them. In order to filter out tweets concerning other topics keywords directly linked to the virus were identified. In 2020, coronavirus was the most searched word on google worldwide. In the US, it came in second place following "election results" (Google Trends, 2020). Similarly., #COVID19 was the most used hashtag on Twitter in 2020 while #StayHome came in third place following #Blacklivesmatter (McGraw, 2020). According to Twitter, the #COVID19 hashtag and "other variations of it" were mentioned approximately 400 million times on Twitter (McGraw, 2020). With the research question in mind it was important to make sure not to exclude tweets written in different variations, especially since the adding of each variation seen above raised the number of tweets appearing in the search. Hence, including them as well as the term pandemic was essential for creating a more comprehensive sample. Moreover, Trump received heavy criticism from the media during this period for often referring to the virus using the terms "China virus", "Chinese virus" and "Chinese plague" (Forgey, 2020, March 18). Looking at tweets containing these terms will help reveal how Trump employed such words. As mentioned before, Trump also made various statements that could be interpreted as promotions for several drugs such as Dexamethasone, Remdesivir, Regeneron, Azithromycin and Hydroxychloroquine (Solender, 2020; Gallagher, 2020). A filtered search with each name revealed Dexamethasone, Remdesivir, Regeneron, Azithromycin did not further the tweets number thus using Hydroxychloroquine as a filtering term revealed all relevant tweets with mentions of drugs.

The World Health Organization had a leading role during this time in facilitating public health strategies while the US Center for Disease Control and Prevention (CDC), the National Institute of Allergy and Infectious Diseases (NIH) and the United States Food and Drug Administration (FDA) play such a leading role within the US. Including tweets related to the three leading organizations as well as Dr. Anthony Fauci, Director of the NIH should help provide new empirical evidence on Trump's language and framing patterns of science and scientists. To better achieve this goal words relating to the main countermeasures recommended by these health organizations such as "social distancing" and "masks" were also used.

## 5.3 Twitter Elements

Percastre-Mendizába et al. (2017), classify elements crucial for understanding political communication on Twitter into three main categories; core variables, input and interactions. Core variables are "highly quantable elements that describe the importance, relevance, presence, and hierarchy of tweeters" (Percastre-Mendizába et al., 2020, p. 582) like an account's number of followers, the number of people followed by the account and the number of retweets and likes received. Until his permanent suspension from Twitter on January 8, 2021, Trump had 88.7 million followers resulting in millions of likes and retweets over the years. In return he only followed 51 accounts mainly owned by his businesses or family members (Mint, 2020, January 9). Since he joined Twitter in 2009, Trump tweeted 56,571 times around 46.4% were published after he was sworn into office on January 20, 2017 (Trump Archiver, January 8).

A Twitter user can share two kinds of inputs; original tweets or retweets. Original tweets refer to tweets containing input that has been directly posted from the tweeter's account (Percastre-Mendizába et al., 2017). Within the context of this paper, the word tweet only refers to original tweets which are those shared directly by @realDonaldTrump using his own language, choice of words as well as construction meaning. Retweets are defined as "original posts repeated and forwarded by another user in order to propagate news" (Wasike , 2013, p. 9). They are usually identified through the presence of the abbreviation RT before the start of the input message (Waiske, 2020). For example, user A sees an original tweet posted by Twitter user B and would like to share it on their own Twitter feed. Twitter provides User A through retweeting with the opportunity to make the original tweet posted by user B available for their own followers. The retweeting function is perceived as a "more passive and less demanding form of engaging with users on social media" (Enli, 2017, p. 54). However, due to its limitations, this paper will only focus on analyzing tweets because they reflect Trump's own communication style.

The third category could be recognized as a subcategory of inputs given that its elements are usually embedded within tweets. It consists of elements made available by Twitter to "interact with and establish relationships with other tweeters" which are hashtags, mentions and shared links (Percastre-Mendizába et al., 2017, p. 582). Although hashtags are now being used on all kinds of social media platforms, they actually originated from Twitter in 2007 (Zhang, 2019). Placing the # sign before a word or a phrase within a tweet while leaving no space between the alphabets or the numbers, results in the creation of a hashtag. These are usually used to organize discussions based on keywords and help track content related to the topic by conducting just one search for the hashtag (Hemphill et al., 2013). Mentions are created with the use of the @ symbol to make a direct link to another account. They could be seen as an invitation to the mentioned account to join the discussion or an announcement for other users declaring a certain connection between the provided content and the account mentioned (Percastre-Mendizába et al., 2017). If user A mentioned User B, clicking on the mention in user's A tweet will open User's B Twitter account. User B will also be notified by Twitter about being mentioned in a tweet posted by User A. Mentions may also function as a method of referencing and crediting the author of the content shared thus giving credibility and liability to what is being shared. In a sense, the person tweeting is telling the followers: This is who or what you should listen to. On the other hand, one could also mention people to send out criticism to them. This is where the manual qualitative nature of this study comes in handy because it enables a human analysis by carefully examining the meaning of language within its context.

Interaction elements also include what Percastre-Mendizába and et al. (2017) refer to as "shared links". Given that a tweet may contain a maximum of 280 characters or unicode glyphs, users who wish to provide longer content do so by embedding a hyperlink within the tweet (Percastre-Mendizába, 2017). Hyperlinks redirect the user to either external content or other tweets posted on the plattform. Golbeck et al. (2010) found that US congress members mainly used links in their tweets that contain news about themselves thereby turning their Twitter account into a "vehicle of self-promotion". Taking this into consideration, this paper aims to look at how Trump employed interaction elements to discuss the COVID-19 pandemic on Twitter.

## 5.4 Data

The search done using the above-mentioned keywords and time period, generated 332 original tweets. However, 16 of those were deleted after their publication. Since the majority of the deleted tweets were posted again and thus occurred twice in the data, they were filtered out leaving 316 original tweets. Out of those, 30 were connected to other tweets that did not fall within the generated search as they did not include any of the filtering words used. Nevertheless, these were part of a thread that includes at least one of the 30 tweets and are thereby related to them. To clarify, a thread is "series of connected Tweets from one person" that allows users to "provide additional context, an update, or an extended point by connecting multiple Tweets together" given that the maximum capacity of one tweet is limited to 280 characters (Twitter, n.d. b). To better understand the meaning of these 30 tweets and avoid their decontextualization, a separate search with each of the 30 tweets was conducted to collect the complementary pieces that build up the complete thread. This resulted in 32 extra tweets that were added based on their publication date and time to the 316 tweets that appeared in the main search. Thus, the complete data of this study consists of 348 tweets.

## 5.5 Typology

Each tweet found within the generated search builds up a single unit of analysis within the context of this study. Both tweets as well as the use of interaction elements embedded in them were interpreted with the help of a qualitative content analysis. Following Hsieh and Shannon's (2005, p. 1278), a content analysis within the context of this paper is defined as "a research method for the subjective interpretation of the content of text data through the systematic classification process of coding and identifying themes or patterns". Hence, it enables researchers to go beyond mere words quantification towards deeper interpretations of the function of words within their context with the help of classifying large materials into clear structured categories (Weber, 1990; Cassel & Symon, 1994). Moreover, it is argued that nuances of political communication could be better captured with the help of qualitative methods given that they are usually explicitly transmitted (Denk, 2011). In this case, a qualitative approach helps researchers to "capture the meanings embedded in the internal relations within texts, which collapsing into reductive measures would obscure." (Reese, 2007, p.10).

Content analysis can be conducted either inductively or deductively depending on the goal of the study. Deductive approaches to content analysis also referred to by some scholars as directed content analysis are recommended for theory and hypothesis testing research, especially when a conclusive amount of knowledge and scientific research is to be found on the issue from which categories that have been validated by multiple scholars can be extracted and generalized to fit different contexts (Hsieh & Shannon, 2005; Linström & Marais, 2012). While an inductive approach or conventional content analysis are better suited for eliciting knowledge and leading empirical findings about a new emerging phenomenon (Hsieh & Shannon, 2005). A limited amount of studies dealing with political framing patterns of the COVID-19 pandemic, particularly Trump's framing patterns was found at the time when this study was initiated. Those found, as seen in the literature review, focused on communication during early stages of the COVID-19 pandemic. Moreover, since the virus itself and its spread constantly and rapidly evolved over time and with it the different medical, scientific and political responses of health organizations and world leaders, it represented new phenomena each day. By looking at journalistic coverage and political communication of Trump's handling of the COVID-19 pandemic as explained in the background and relevance chapter there could be no denial that it has also presented a new phenomenon of how a US president managed a health crisis, let alone one that in itself represented a new phenomenon within this century (Ladkin, 2020). Thus, an inductive approach was chosen following the recommendation; "If there is not enough former knowledge about the phenomenon or if this knowledge is fragmented, the inductive approach is recommended" (Elo & Kyngäs, 2008, p. 109). In deductive research, categories are predefined and the data is then classified accordingly. The research question is thereby answered through identifying the occurrence of common generic/thematic found in existing scientific research such as conflict frame, the attribution of responsibility frame, the economic consequences frame, and the human-interest frame (Semetko & Valkenburg, 2000). Inductive approaches, on the other hand, require researchers to keep an open view following a ground up strategy that allows categories and their names to emerge from the data (Linström & Marais, 2012). The data was coded entirely manually in order to be able to interpret "cultural, linguistic, or latent meanings during the coding and analysis that may be missed by computerized analysis" (Foley et al., 2019, p. 1814). This is mainly based on the argument that "a frame has a certain pattern in a given text" composed of elements grouped together in a specific way that triggers a certain line of interpretation (Matthes & Kohring, 2008). Thus, rather than coding abstract frames, analytical units are broken down into elements that are coded and interpreted along the content analysis procedure. Before doing that, the data was entirely gone through at once to achieve a sense of the whole and repeated to achieve full immersion (Tesch, 2013). This was followed by an in-depth word to word reading to identify and underline framing patterns.

D'Angelo and Kuypers (2010, p. 91) argue that frames are "packages" of organizing ideas constructed through the exclusion, inclusion or salience of manifest elements in the text referred to as framing devices. Framing devices were classified into three different categories; First, rhetorical devices which represent language tools found on the textual level such as keywords, metaphors, catchphrases, exemplars, spins, contrasts (Gamson and Modigliani, 1989). While these are usually explicitly present in the unit of analysis, reasoning devices are more implicit elements and may not always be visually or technically identifiable in text for researchers to merely point at (Gamson and Modigliani, 1989). However, the presence and denotation of the rhetorical devices may implicitly put forward a certain line of argumentation that defines the issue and its roots, give justifications and possibly suggest interpretations and solutions (Entman, 1993). Thereby, reasoning devices rest on the defying functions of frames presented in the theory chapter and demonstrate how the different frame elements come together to "form a route of causal reasoning which may be evoked when an issue is associated with a particular frame" (Van Gorp, 2010, p. 91). The third set of framing devices constituted technical devices. In traditional news media analysis, researchers try to interpret how content is being highlighted through tools such headlines, subheadlines, visual elements as well as sources and quotations (Reese et al., 2003). Given that the medium of this study is Twitter the above-mentioned interaction elements represented in hashtags, mentions and hyperlinks were added as they represent the new form of technical devices on Twitter. However, just like in traditional media, quotes and sources remain strong framing devices since they are used to add credibility, validity as well as facticity or authoritativeness to the given argument or line of interpretation (Reese et al., 2003). As follows, this paper examined how Trump used Twitter's technical devices to support and convey his pattern of framing to the public. It should be noted that pictures and videos were excluded as visual framing falls beyond the scope of this paper. The previous steps were followed through an open coding of the text. Tweet elements were broken down and illustrated visually within a matrix developed for each tweet. Each row encompasses the different elements found in one tweet while each column is a distinction between the types of elements. This was done to bring a systematic overview on what framing devices come together to form a framing pattern. In this way, the researcher was able to compare patterns of devices and connect them to overreaching ideas. Thereby, also highlighting similarities, differences and contrasts between the tweets and the frames they carry (Van Gorp, 2010). The goal was to search for logical combinations across the columns such as problem definition, causal responsibility, solutions, treatment responsibility (Entman, 1993). A compact visual illustration of the analysis procedure is reflected in Figure 1:

**Figure 1**

*Methodology*

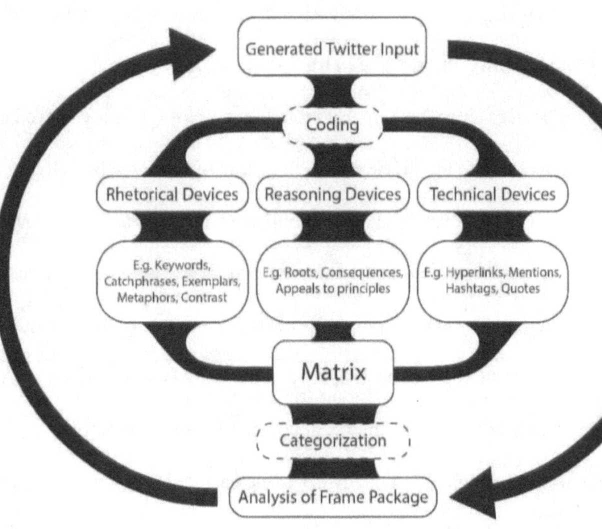

# 6 Results

## 6.1 Epidemic (January 24 – March 10, 2020)

"It will all work out well" (Trump, 2020, January 24)

Between January 24 and March 10, 2020, Trump tweets were mainly focused on reassuring the public that the "Coronavirus is very much under control in the USA" (Trump, 2020, February 24). The name "Coronavirus" was mostly used, however Trump also referred to it using general and undefined names like "a virus" or "the virus" (e.g., Trump, 2020, February 7b, January 24). Only on March 3, 2020 did he include China in his naming of the Coronavirus by referring to it as "China's Coronavirus", thereby clearly identifying China as the source of the virus. Trump (2020, February 28a) also indicated that China is to blame because the coronavirus "started in China and spread to various countries throughout the world". However, up until that point Trump framed China as a cooperative partner that is in close connection with the US (e.g., Trump, 2020, January 24, 27, 30). In his very first tweet from January 24, 2020 Trump even said: "The United States greatly appreciates their efforts and transparency" and portrayed China as a very hard-working country that is doing its best "to contain" the Coronavirus (Trump, 2020, January 24). Thus, war metaphors were used to describe the situation in China and portray the Chinese President as a "strong, sharp and powerfully focused" hero that is leading a "counterattack on the Coronavirus" and a "very successful operation" (Trump, 2020, February 7a).

At the same time, the coronavirus epidemic in the US was defined as a non-threatening "situation" (e.g., February 27a, March 5a, March 9a) that might even go away especially "as the weather starts to warm & the virus hopefully becomes weaker, and then gone" (Trump, 2020, February 7b). Similarly, by saying: "If the virus disappeared tomorrow", there is an activation of the idea that the situation is temporary and that there is a possibility that the contagious disease might just vanish (Trump, 2020, February 25b). When talking about the consequences of the coronavirus in the US, Trump focused on presenting a positive picture, highlighting America's exceptionalism and presenting the numbers of infections and deaths in the country as being very low especially in comparison to other countries (e.g. Trump, 2020, February 24, February 28a, March 5b). The reason offered by Trump for why the US is "way ahead" of other countries (Trump, 2020, February 28b) is reflected in the following tweet:

> So, the Coronavirus, which started in China and spread to various countries throughout the world, but very slowly in the U.S. because President Trump closed our border, and ended flights, VERY EARLY,is now being blamed, by the Do Nothing Democrats, to be the fault of "Trump". (Trump, 2020, February 28a)

Thus, border and flight closing were presented as the most appropriate treatment recommendation. The very early closing of the borders is particularly emphasized, as indicated by the capitalization in this tweet, and which was also described by Trump in another tweet as a "Godsend" (Trump, 2020, March 8).

Meanwhile, immigrants were pictured as a threat by distinguishing between the source of coronavirus cases in the US based on nationality:

> With approximately 100,000 CoronaVirus cases worldwide, and 3,280 deaths, the United States, because of quick action on closing our borders, has, as of now, only 129 cases (40 Americans brought in) and 11 deaths. We are working very hard to keep these numbers as low as possible! (Trump, 2020, March 5b)

In that way, blame was put on the foreigners or the 'others' thus drawing a picture of us vs. them. The Democrat Party, also referred to as the "Do Nothing Democrats" or "Dems" (e.g. Trump, 2020, February 28b), and the Media under the name "Fake News Media" (e.g. Trump, 2020, March 8), were framed as partners who are only exaggerating the "situation" and putting out "disinformation" with the goal of harming him personally and undermining "the incredible & successful effort being made!" (Trump, 2020, March 5c, March 9a). Both the media and the Democratic Party were accused of politicizing the epidemic. Meanwhile, Trump framed himself as their victim using words like "Not fair" and "Sad" and portrayed himself as the one who knows better through putting out assertions like "Dems called it VERY wrong!" or "I was right. He is incompetent!" referring to democratic senator Chuck Schumer who he named "Cryin' Chuck Schumer" (Trump, 2020, February 25a, March 8).

Nonetheless, during the first epidemic period Trump tweets carried a positive framing pattern towards health professionals and experts. For example, Trump said "CDC & World Health have been working hard and very smart" on February 24, 2020.

However, praising and crediting health professionals for their effort was also done through hyperbolic language that reinforced a narrative of America's exceptionalism. For example: "We have the best experts anywhere in the world, and they are on top of it 24/7!" (Trump, 2020, January 29).

During this period, no appeals were made to the public on how to deal with the "situation" or prevent the spread of the coronavirus. Indeed, Trump's only appeal was to think about the difference between the number of Americans who have died from the common Flu compared to the number of confirmed Coronavirus cases. In this way, Trump further downplayed the coronavirus by comparing it to the common Flu and even evaluated it as a less lethal disease as indicated in the following tweet published only two days before the WHO characterized COVID-19 as a pandemic:

> So last year 37,000 Americans died from the common Flu. It averages between 27,000 and 70,000 per year. Nothing is shut down, life & the economy go on. At this moment there are 546 confirmed cases of CoronaVirus, with 22 deaths. Think about that! (Trump, 2020, March 9b)

### 6.2 Pandemic (March 11 – September 28, 2020)

"THE CURE CANNOT BE WORSE (by far) THAN THE PROBLEM!" (Trump, 2020, March 24)

Between March 11 and September 28, 2020 Trump's tweets were mainly focused on downplaying the threat of the pandemic, deflecting blame, sending out hopeful messages, pushing to open the economy, portraying America as the "Greatest

Country in the world" (Trump, 2020, March 11a), praising himself and his administration's work, using the COVID-19 pandemic to campaign for his reelection, and issuing attacks on the Democratic party, China, the media, the Obama Administration, the WHO, the FDA, as well health experts such as Dr. Anthony Fauci.

Various names were used to refer to the coronavirus including the "Chinese virus", "China virus", "Covid", "Covid-19", "plague", 'China's plague", "the invisible virus", the invisible enemy" and "the virus" (e.g. Trump, 2020, May 16, May 20, June 30, July 27, September 16). Although Trump continuously undermined the real threat of the COVID-19 pandemic, there was a shift towards more seriousness in his tone in comparison to the first period. The term "situation" was still used to refer to the COVID-19 pandemic however new terms such as a "challenge" and "a problem" appeared (e.g. Trump, 2020, March 11c, March 12). He also resorted to using war metaphors by using terms such as "battle", "onslaught", "defeat", "beat", "victory", "win", "survive", "marshalling", "fighting" and "hit" (e.g. Trump, 2020, March 18a, March 27, May 1, August 11). On March 11, 2020, Trump published a tweet that was fully dominated by the war frame in terms of problem definition, moral evaluation, and appeals to the public, thereby portraying himself as a wartime President:

> The Media should view this as a time of unity and strength. We have a common enemy, actually, an enemy of the World, the CoronaVirus. We must beat it as quickly and safely as possible. There is nothing more important to me than the life & safety of the United States! (Trump, 2020, March 11b)

Beside directly linking China to the coronavirus by using various name variations, Trump continuously framed China as the cause and origin of the COVID-19 pandemic (e.g. Trump, 2020, May 16, May 20, June 30, September 8, September 30). One of the most explicit references to this can be seen in his tweet from May 28, 2020, in which he described the coronavirus as "a very bad 'gift' from China". Nearly one month before that, Trump defended his naming politics by saying that "it did start with 'one person from China', and then grew, & will be a 'Miracle' end!" (Trump, 2020, April 25). In his tweet from June 30, 2020, Trump very obviously employed the language of fear and anger towards China:

> As I watch the Pandemic spread its ugly face all across the world, including the tremendous damage it has done to the USA, I become more and more angry at China. People can see it, and I can feel it! (Trump, 2020, June 30)

Through this tweet, Trump makes appeals to the American people to see China as the cause of their suffering and encourages them to feel anger towards China. Those who fail to do so, such as the Democrats and the media, were blamed and insulted for failing. For example, Trump wrote:

> So now the Fake News @nytimes is tracing the CoronaVirus origins back to Europe, NOT China. This is a first! I wonder what the Failing New York Times got for this one? Are there any NAMED sources? They were recently thrown out of China like dogs, and obviously want back in. Sad! (Trump, 2020, April 11).

At the same time, Trump accused CBS and its show 60 Minutes for trying to do everything "to defend China and the horrible Virus pandemic that was inflicted on the USA and the rest of the World. I guess they want to do business in China!" (Turmp, 2020, May 10b). The use of the word inflicted further reinforces an image of China as a villain who actively and intentionally caused the US and the world harm. The Democrats were also accused of falling "to blame their cash cow, China, for the plague." (Trump, 2020, May 2). Moreover, the image of China as a cooperative partner and a hard-working country that is doing its best "to contain" the coronavirus and being transparent (Trump, 2020, January 24) was transformed into an incompetent and reckless enemy who "could have easily stopped the plague" but didn't (Trump, 2020, May 20). Thus, Trump continued to present his very early closing of the borders and entry from China as a solution without which many more lives would have been lost (e.g. Trump, 2020, March 13a, April 7). The language of xenophobia and fear of immigrants dominated many of the tweets throughout this phase. For example, Trump wrote: "To this point, and because we have had a very strong border policy, we have had 40 deaths related to CoronaVirus. If we had weak or open borders, that number would be many times higher!" (Trump, 2020, March 13a). Moreover, Trump directly linked his plan to construct a wall along the US borders with Mexico to the COVID-19 pandemic by presenting it as a positive strategy to combat the spread of the coronavirus in the US:

> Mexico is sadly experiencing very big CoronaVirus problems, and now California, get this, doesn't want people coming over the Southern Border. A

> Classic! They are sooo lucky that I am their President. Border is very tight and the Wall is rapidly being built! (Trump, 2020, May 4)

All this came in contrast to a tweet published earlier in which he called to protect the Asian community from xenophobia and blame:

> It is very important that we totally protect our Asian American community in the United States, and all around the world. They are amazing people, and the spreading of the Virus is NOT their fault in any way, shape, or form. They are working closely with us to get rid of it. WE WILL PREVAIL TOGETHER! (Trump, 2020, March 23b)

While stressing border closings as a solution, Trump did not see lockdowns as a helpful nor necessary solution for protecting the public health. Thus, he promoted for easing measures by arguing that:

> Our people want to return to work. They will practice Social Distancing and all else, and Seniors will be watched over protectively & lovingly. We can do two things together. THE CURE CANNOT BE WORSE (by far) THAN THE PROBLEM! Congress MUST ACT NOW. We will come back strong! (Trump, 2020, March 24)

Through messages like this, Trump placed himself on the side of the workers against the political elite who was depriving the people from their work and refusing to act quickly in their favor. Meanwhile, he also painted a rosy picture of the economy and the future while using lockdown measures to campaign against his political rival Joe Biden (e.g. Trump, 2020, June 25, July, 8, September 10). For example, he wrote "Coronavirus deaths are way down. Mortality rate is one of the lowest in the World. Our Economy is roaring back and will NOT be shut down. "Embers" or flare ups will be put out, as necessary!" (Trump, 2020, June 25). Similarly, he argued that:

> Sleepy Joe Biden, the puppet of the Left, ever won. Markets would crash and cities would burn. Our Country would suffer like never before. We will beat the Virus, soon, and go on to the Golden Age - better than ever before! (Trump, 2020, July 27)

As seen above, during this period, there was a focus on showing that everything is under control and that the threat of the COVID-19 pandemic is decreasing with mortality rate and infection numbers going down, due to his successful response (e.g. Trump, 2020, July 6a, July 7). Only once did Trump speak about the number of COVID-19 infections using a negative tone while recognizing its human impact on society:

> We have just reached a very sad milestone with the coronavirus pandemic deaths reaching 100,000. To all of the families & friends of those who have passed, I want to extend my heartfelt sympathy & love for everything that these great people stood for & represent. God be with you!

Otherwise, the rise of the infection number was continuously framed as a result of the best coronavirus testing system in the world. The media and the Democratic Party were still being framed as partners but also as a "Hoax" (Trump, April 25, 2020). Both sides were accused of exaggerating the pandemic threat and politicizing the pandemic to undermine his successful handling of the COVID-19 pandemic. For example:

> The only reason the U.S. has reported one million cases of CoronaVirus is that our Testing is sooo much better than any other country in the World. Other countries are way behind us in Testing, and therefore show far fewer cases! (Trump, 2020, April 29)

> The Radical Left Lamestream Media, together with their partner, the Do Nothing Democrats, are trying to spread a new narrative that President Trump was slow in reacting to Covid 19. Wrong, I was very fast, even doing the Ban on China long before anybody thought necessary! (Trump, 2020, May 27)

Beside referring to them as the "Do Nothing Democrats", Trump framed the Democrats as incompetent "radical left" complainers and liars who are just looking to personally harm him by inflaming the COVID-19 pandemic situation (Trump, 2020, August 7). Phrases like "RUDE and NASTY", "heartless", "angry", "always, looking for trouble" and that they do "nothing constructive, even in times of crisis" were employed to further draw an image of Democratic politicians as part of the political elite that does not have the public's best interest in mind (Trump, 2020, April 18, May 2, September 16). Trump also issued personal attacks on Democratic politicians including Joe Biden (e.g. Sleepy Joe, corrupt Joe Biden), Nancy Pelosi (Crazy Nancy), Chuck Schumer, Barack Obama and Andrew Cuomo (e.g. Trump, 2020, May 26, June 27). Undermining and attacking Democrats was also carried out by repeatedly using the same exemplar. Exemplars help frame issues using stories for example, historical examples, myths, or legends from which one can learn a lesson. They function as bridges between the present and the past (Gamson & Modigliani, 1989). Trump drew a connection between the coronavirus and the H1N1 Swine Flu to accuse the Obama Administration including his 2020 election rival Joe Biden for failing to handle the H1N1 pandemic in 2009 and praise himself and his administration for doing a much better job (e.g. Trump 2020, March 15a, May 10a, September 3). He wanted the public to think of them as the "Gang That Couldn't Shoot Straight", which by implicit contrast means that he is the one who can. In a similar vein, he wrote:

> We are getting great marks for the handling of the CoronaVirus pandemic, especially the very early BAN of people from China, the infectious source, entering the USA. Compare that to the Obama/Sleepy Joe disaster known as H1N1 Swine Flu. Poor marks, bad polls - didn't have a clue! (Trump, 2020, May 10a)

Another historical exemplar was used to argue against Mail-In-Ballots and accuse Democrats of "[u]sing Covid to steal the state" (Trump, 2020, August 3a). Trump compared the COVID-19 Pandemic to World War I and World War II thereby directly activating a war frame and turning a health crisis into a political issue:

> Because of MAIL-IN BALLOTS, 2020 will be the most RIGGED Election in our nations history - unless this stupidity is ended. We voted during World War One

> & World War Two with no problem, but now they are using Covid in order to cheat by using Mail-Ins! (Trump, 2020, June 22a)

Trump made comparisons to other countries to highlight America's exceptionalism and self-praise himself for the "VERY high marks" of his administration's work compared to other countries (Trump, 2020, September 7). To further reinforce this narrative, Trump proudly announced donations to other countries and presented their situation as being much worse than in the US (e.g. Trump, 2020, March 12, May 15, April 24, July 21a, August 3b). He also used comparisons to indicate that he took the right decisions:

> Sweden is paying heavily for its decision not to lockdown. As of today, 2462 people have died there, a much higher number than the neighboring countries of Norway (207), Finland (206) or Denmark (443). The United States made the correct decision! (Trump, 2020, April 30)

Two main solutions, besides closed borders and travel bans were mentioned several times: First, Hydroxychloroquine as a beneficial drug that could help mitigate the effects of the coronavirus and even when taken with Azithromycin "have a real chance to be one of the biggest game changers in the history of medicine" (Trump, 2020, March 21). The only time Trump relied on a scientific health study was to argue for the effectiveness of Hydroxychloroquine:

> The highly respected Henry Ford Health System just reported, based on a large sampling, that HYDROXYCHLOROQUINE cut the death rate in certain sick patients very significantly. The Dems disparaged it for political reasons (me!). Disgraceful. Act now @US_FDA @TuckerCarlson @FoxNews (Trump, 2020, July 6b).

Governmental agencies were also ordered to "MOVE FAST" in their acceptance process of Hydroxychloroquine. The second discussed solution was: vaccines and therapeutics mentioned together (e.g. Trump, 2020, May 6, June 2, July 15, July 21b). The development of vaccines was framed as an American success that further makes the country better than the rest of the world also using hyperbolic language to describe the progress (e.g., Trump, 2020, July 21a). On September 25, Trump clearly said: "Vaccines are being developed by the finest Labs in the World." (Trump, 2020, September 25)

However, the FDA was accused of hindering the process for political reasons. In this way, Trump framed the governmental health agency as being against him and against the public's interest. He even evoked a line of conspiracy theory by calling the FDA the "deep state":

> The deep state, or whoever, over at the FDA is making it very difficult for drug companies to get people in order to test the vaccines and therapeutics. Obviously, they are hoping to delay the answer until after November 3rd. Must focus on speed, and saving lives! @SteveFDA (Trump, 2020, August 22)

The CDC was also criticized for failing to prepare for a large-scale pandemic thereby deflecting blame on the agency (e.g. Trump, 2020, March 13b). Moreover, the opinion of Dr. Anthony Fauci, NIH Director Member of the White House Coronavirus Task force was framed as irrelevant in a tweet in which Trump deliberately said that he "Informed Dr. Fauci this morning that he has nothing to do with NFL Football." (Trump, 2020, June 19) referring to suggestions made by Fauci to avoid football games in the Fall due to the rise of COVID-19 infections (Alvarado, 2020, June 20). Trump also tried to deflect blame onto the WHO in three tweets from April 7 and April 17, 2020 in which he accused the organization of making several "inaccurate or misleading" claims and having a delayed response to the COVID-19 pandemic. On April 7, 2020 Trump framed his own decisions as being better that the WHO's recommendations:

> The W.H.O. really blew it. For some reason, funded largely by the United States, yet very China centric. We will be giving that a good look. Fortunately I rejected their advice on keeping our borders open to China early on. Why did they give us such a faulty recommendation? (Trump, 2020, April 7)

However, Trump praised US health professionals and experts in general using hyperbolic language that speaks to his idea of America being better than the other countries: "America is the Greatest Country in the world. We have the best scientists, doctors, nurses and health care professionals. They are amazing people who do phenomenal things every day" (Trump, 2020, March 11a)

From March 11 to 28 September, 2020 Trump made appeals to the public to socially distance only three times (Trump, 2020, March 14a, March 19, April 9), while suggesting wearing masks only once during the entire period, only because it is something that is being viewed as a "Patriotic" act. In this way, wearing a mask is portrayed as a sacrifice he is willing to make, for the good of the nation:

> We are United in our effort to defeat the Invisible China Virus, and many people say that it is Patriotic to wear a face mask when you can't socially distance yourself. There is nobody more Patriotic than me, your favorite President!

Moreover, catchphrases like: "Together we will beat the invisible enemy!" (Trump, 2020, March 15b), "Together, we will PREVAIL!", "We will be bigger, better and stronger than ever before!" (Trump, 2002, March 16), "we are all in this TOGETHER!" (Trump, 2020, March 18b) and "Together, we will endure, we will prevail, and we will WIN! (Trump, 2020, March 27) evoke a frame of COVID-19 as a war that can be won, if the nation unites together and follows their heroic leader.

### 6.3 Pre-election Period (29, September - 3 November, 2020)

"This election is a choice between a Trump Super Boom or a Biden Depression, and it's between a safe vaccine or a devastating Biden lockdown!" (Trump, 2020, October 30)

With the start of the first election debate on 29, September 2020, Trump intensified his politicization of the COVID-19 pandemic focusing on attacking his rival Joe Biden, the Democratic Party, the media and lockdowns. His tweets were centered around drawing a positive picture of the US economy and the consequences of the COVID-19 pandemic. He focused on reflecting strength after his infection with COVID-19, thereby minimizing the effect of the coronavirus and defining it as being non-threatening. At the same time, he practiced self-praise and employed exemplars to undermine the Obama administration and contrasts to highlight America's exceptionalism. Similar to the second period, various names were used to refer to the coronavirus including "Chinese virus", "China virus", "Covid", "Covid-19", "plague", "China's plague", "Chinese plague" or "the virus" (Trump, 2020, September 29, September 30, October 5). However, no mention of the "invisible enemy" or "invisible virus" were made during this period. His use of war related terminology also remained limited to "fighting", "hit job" and a "battle" (Trump, 2020, October 3, October 6, October 12).

When announcing his own infection with COVID-19, Trump said "We will get through this TOGETHER!", thereby seeking the public's empathy and including them as part of his personal life. Shortly before his release from the hospital, he made a clear statement that downplayed the Coronavirus threat and portrayed him as being unshaken and unharmed with no consideration to the more than 200,000 thousand lives lost to the coronavirus in the US and their families (see appendix). "Don't let it dominate your life. We have developed, under the Trump Administration, some really great drugs & knowledge. I feel better than I did 20 years ago!" (Trump, 2020, October 5). With the use of hyperbole of feeling better than 20 years ago, Trump made sure to erase any doubt about the virus having even the slightest negative effect on him. To further reinforce his argument, Trump compared COVID-19 to the common Flu to use it as an argument to ease lockdown measures:

> Flu season is coming up! Many people every year, sometimes over 100,000, and despite the Vaccine, die from the Flu. Are we going to close down our Country? No, we have learned to live with it, just like we are learning to live with Covid, in most populations far less lethal!!! (Trump, 2020, October 6)

Meanwhile, Trump used his infection with COVID-19 to praise his Administration and frame it as a successful solution finder while referring to himself in third person. Nonetheless, he remained consistent on framing China as the source and cause of the spread of COVID-19: "It wasn't their fault that the Plague came in from China! Democrat cities and states" (Trump, 2020, October 21). On October 27, the virus was personified using a metaphor that is connected to immigration by saying: "The fact is that we have learned and done a lot about this Virus. Much different now than when it first arrived on our shores, and the World's, from China!" (Trump, 2020, October 27a), thus, framing the coronavirus as a foreign threat and further emphasizing border closings as a solution that the Democrats wouldn't be able to deliver: "My highly regarded Executive Order protected 525,000 American jobs during the height of the Chinese Plague. Democrats want to have Open Borders! (Trump, 2020, October 7)". Meanwhile, his framing attacks on the media continued because they are just "very bad (and sick!) people!" (Trump, 2020, October 13) who are using the pandemic to harm him before elections:

> We have made tremendous progress with the China Virus, but the Fake News refuses to talk about it this close to the Election. COVID, COVID, COVID is being used by them, in total coordination, in order to change our great early election numbers.Should be an election law violation! (Trump, 2020, October 26)

Due to the nearing of the elections, Trump focused during this period on drawing a binary picture of black-and-white while denouncing the negative consequences that will follow if he is no longer America's president. Lockdowns were weaponized as a method to attack Biden by focusing on the economic drawbacks of lockdown policies rather than the public health issue.

> This election is a choice between a TRUMP RECOVERY or a BIDEN DEPRESSION. It's a choice between a TRUMP BOOM or a BIDEN LOCKDOWN. It's a choice between our plan to Kill the virus – or Biden's plan to kill the American Dream! (Trump, 2020, October 27b)

Hence, the main solution offered during this period to overcome the COVID-19 pandemic was to vote for him. His tweets about the COVID-19 pandemic during this period were used as a campaigning method and thus rather focused on the economy and making promises with the help of a highly positive hyperbolic language to project hope into a future with him as the leader: "We are leading the World in Economic Recovery, and THE BEST IS YET TO COME!" (Trump, 2020, October 6). Vaccines were also as an upcoming solution but the FDA is framed as standing in the way of making that happen out of political reasons (e.g. Trump, 2020, October 6).

Trump also continued to use the situation to denounce the Democratic Party and its candidate Joe Biden. To do this he used the same H1N1 swine Flu exemplar to argue that Biden is incompetent and won't be able to with the use of insulting language:

> Joe Biden's response to the H1N1 Swine Flu, far less lethal than Covid 19, was one of the weakest and worst in the history of fighting epidemics and pandemics. It was pathetic, those involved have said. Joe didn't have a clue! (Trump, 2020, October 23)

No appeals to the public were made regarding social distancing or wearing masks. The main appeal was to vote for Trump on election day because "The great American Comeback is underway!!!" (Trump, 2020, November 1)

### 6.4 Post-Election Period (November 4, 2020 - January 8, 2021)

"Our Country, and indeed the World, will soon see the great miracle of what the Trump Administration has accomplished" (Trump, 2020, December 22)

After election day, Trump's main focus was on vaccines. His tweets mainly focused on praising himself and his administration for the successful development of vaccines in the US, one that could not have been achieved under any other Administration. All framing devices were employed to serve this goal or attack the media and Joe Biden. The coronavirus was mainly referred to as the "China virus", "Covid", "Covid-19" and "China's plague" (e.g., Trump, 2020, November 16, November 21, December 9, January 3).

Trump's tweets throughout this period were explicitly aimed at ensuring that he only gets the credit for the development of the vaccines: "Another Vaccine just announced. This time by Moderna, 95% effective. For those great "historians", please remember that these great discoveries, which will end the China Plague, all took place on my watch!" (Trump, 2020, November 16)

Meanwhile, science and health institutions especially the FDA, were given no credit at all but instead undermined, insulted and accused of politicizing the vaccine approval process:

> While my pushing the money drenched but heavily bureaucratic @US_FDA saved five years in the approval of NUMEROUS great new vaccines, it is still a big, old, slow turtle. Get the dam vaccines out NOW, Dr. Hahn @SteveFDA. Stop playing games and start saving lives!!! (Trump, 2020, December 11a, see also November 9, November 30)

Trump issued a similar accusation towards Democrats and the vaccine development company, Pfizer, arguing that they deliberately delayed the approval process for after election day in order to deprive him of the success he might receive because of that:

> As I have long said, @Pfizer and the others would only announce a Vaccine after the Election, because they didn't have the courage to do it before. Likewise, the @US_FDA should have announced it earlier, not for political purposes, but for saving lives! (Trump, 2020, November 9)

In addition to attaching China to the name of the coronavirus, Trump also identified the "China Virus", in particular, as the cause of the American people suffering: "$2000 for our great people, not $600! They have suffered enough from the China Virus!!!" (Trump, 2020, December 29) thereby directly inflicting blame of China. At the same time, during this period, the media continued to be subjected to accusation for failing to report the truth while exaggerating the effects of the COVID-19 pandemic in the US in order to personally harm him: "Fake News always "forgets" to mention that far fewer people are dying when they get Covid. This is do to both our advanced therapeutics, and the gained knowledge of our great doctors, nurses and front line workers!" (Trump 2020, November 21)

Different comparisons to other countries were made with the same goal of portraying an image of the US as being ahead of other countries. For example: "Europe and other parts of the World being hit hard by the China Virus - Germany, France, Spain and Italy, in particular. The vaccines are on their way!!!" (Trump, 2020, December 18)

The main difference, in this period, is Trump's framing of the US as the savior of the world because of vaccine development.

> The entire WORLD is being badly hurt by the China Virus, but if you listen to the Fake News Lamestream Media, and Big Tech, you would think that we are the only one. No, but we are the Country that developed vaccines, and years ahead of schedule! (Trump, 2020, December 19)

No appeals were made to the public during this period, except to watch out for possible election fraud: "WATCH FOR MASSIVE BALLOT COUNTING ABUSE AND, JUST LIKE THE EARLY VACCINE, REMEMBER I TOLD YOU SO!" (Trump, 2020, November 10)

## 6.5 Mentions

Throughout the entire study period Trump made 113 mentions. The most mentioned account belonged to the US Food and Drug Administration with a total of 10 mentions. However, Trump used two different accounts to refer to the FDA; 7 times using the correct official Twitter account (@US_FDA) and 3 times using the tag of an inactive account that redirects the user to the official account (@FDA). The FDA was mainly mentioned by Trump to be given orders to by using phrases such as: "Act now @US_FDA" (Trump, 2020, July 6b) and "@FDA move quickly!" (Trump, 2020, September 23) or criticized e.g. "The @US_FDA and the Democrats didn't want to have me get a Vaccine WIN, prior to the election" (Trump, 2020, November 9). Only once did Trump mention the FDA to thank them for their work: "The FDA has moved mountains - Thank You!" (Trump, 2020, March 21). Similarly, the FDA commissioner during Trump's presidency, Stephen Hahn, was mentioned 4 times, once to be thanked and three times to be criticized e.g. "Dr. Hahn @SteveFDA Stop playing games and start saving lives!!!" (Trump, 2020, December 11). The US Center for Disease Control and Prevention was mentioned 7 times (@CDCgov). In two instances during the first period, Trump refers to the organization using a positive tone of praise and appreciation e.g.

"@CDCgov, @SecAzar and all doing a great job with respect to Coronavirus!" (Trump, 2020, February 26). The other mentions were either deployed to give order to or criticize the CDC e.g. "For decades the @CDCgov looked at, and studied, its testing system, but did nothing about it." (Trump, 2020, March 13).

Fox News was mentioned in 6 tweets while Trish Regan, a conservative Fox News media host was mentioned twice for the same purpose of redistributing content or quotes that originated from the news outlet and its staff and had a positive sentiment towards Trump or his administration or a negative sentiment towards other news outlets or the Democratic Party. For example: "His (President Trump's) policies set a foundation that allowed us to survive the pandemic." @HeyTammyBruce @SteveHiltonx @FoxNews True, we built something so strong that we are now setting economic growth records again - Jobs & Growth!!! (Trump, 2020, June 22b)

> "Diagnosis positive: @CNN is infected with Trump Derangement Syndrome. I'm calling out CNN for irresponsibly politicizing what should be a unifying battle against a virus that doesn't choose sides." @trish_regan @FoxNews Like I say, they are Fake News! (Trump, 2020, February 27b)

Breitbart News was also mentioned twice to reinforce and redistribute content posted by the Network. For example: "Report: Maryland Gov. Larry Hogan, Anti-Trump Hero, Paid for Flawed Coronavirus Tests from South Korea https://t.co/PHV7euutVb via @BreitbartNews." (Trump, 2020, November 22). On the other hand, CNN, The New York Times and 60 Minutes the news magazine broadcast from CBS News were each mentioned 3 times to be attacked and criticized. For example, “Fake News @CNN” and “Fake News @nytimes” (Trump, 2020, April 11, April 22).

Only three Twitter accounts of non-American political actors were mentioned by President Trump in three distinctive tweets: Canadian Prime Minister Justin Trudeau, Indian Prime Minister Narenda Modi and the Prime Minister of the United Kingdom Boris Johnson. All three tweets were written with a positive attitude to reflect having a cooperative relationship with the Primes Ministers and their respective countries. Prime Minister Johnson was thanked by President Trump “for his friendship and support” and described as a "great guy”. Meanwhile, Prime Minister Modi was mentioned to be given support to by President Trump or perhaps his administration, considering the use of the word “we” not “I”: “We stand with India and @narendramodi during this pandemic.” The Canadian Prime Minister was mentioned in a tweet after the two “[j]ust had a nice conversation” - to announce that “[t]he United States and Canada will continue to coordinate closely together on COVID-19.” (Trump, 2020, March 14b). Trump’s Vice President Mike Pence and his Secretary of Health and Human Services, as well Republican Governor of Ohio Mike DeWine were mentioned to either be thanked or praised for their work (**Fehler! Verweisquelle konnte nicht gefunden werden.**).

**Figure 2**

*Mention Frequency in Tweets*

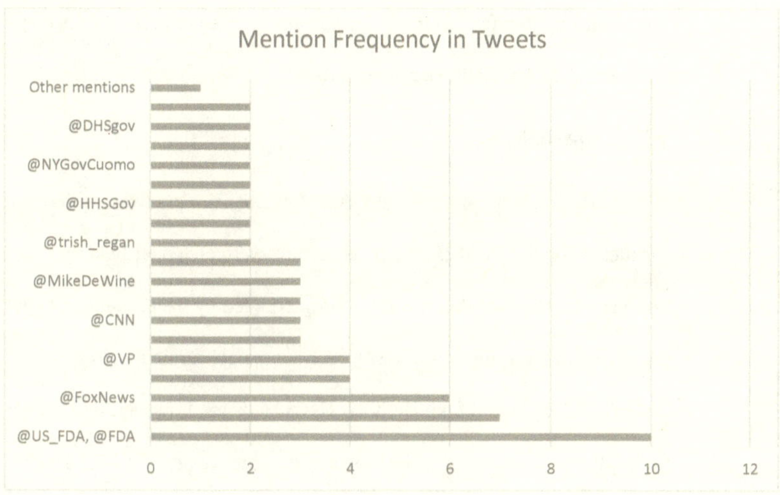


## 6.6 Quotes

Quotes were mainly used by Trump as a technical framing device to reinforce voices that praise him or his administration's work. The majority of the quotes originated from Fox News personalities and Republican politicians like Trish Regan, Maria Bartiromo, Ronny Jackson, Tammy Bruce and Steve Hilton. For example, on March 5, 2020 Trump shared a quote from Republican Senator Tom Cotton: "I want to commend the President for how he has handled the CoronaVirus situation, especially his early decision to shut down access into our Country from China, despite strong opposition to that decision." (Trump, 2020, March 5d)

Similarly, on December 11, 2020 a quote from Fox Business Network talk show Varney & Co. was used to reinforce an image of vaccines as a "miracle" that Trump should be credited for: "Donald Trump must get the credit for the vaccines. It is a miracle." (Trump, 2020, December 11b)

### 6.7 Hyperlinks

The majority of hyperlinks shared within Trump's tweets referred back to his own Twitter account. Since his twitter account was suspended on January 8, 2021. The links were unavailable and thus could not be interpreted by the researcher. Other links shared by Trump had varying sources with each source appearing maximum once. Two Hyperlinks originated from Breitbart News Network, however, the number still remains insignificant. Thus, no interpretation could be put forward on what source was mainly relied on. Since analyzing the content of the links falls out of the scope of the paper the following table should provide an overview of the sources that appeared in the data.

**Table 1**

*Quote by Source*

| News Outlets (13) | Journalists (5) | Politicians (2) |
|---|---|---|
| Breitbart News (2) | Mark Knoller / CBS News (1) | Ronna McDanie / GOP Chairwoman (1) |
| Fox News (1) | Allan Smith / NBC News (1) | Mike Pence / Vice President (1) |
| ITV News (1) | Ciarán Ó Fathaigh / AbandonedBerlin (Link to APNews) (1) | Trump (16) |
| National Review (1) | Paige Southwick Pfleger / WOSU Public Media (1) | Trump Twitter account (13) |
| NBC News (1) | Pat St. Claire / Wabe.org (Link to CNN) (1) | Team Trump Twitter account (3) |
| New York Post (1) | Gov. Sources (4) | |
| Old Life (1) | The White House 45 Archived (2) | |
| The Dallas Morning News (1) | CDC (1) | |
| The Hill (1) | Stephen M. Hahn / Former FDA Comissioner (1) | |
| The New York Times (1) | | |
| The Washington Times (1) | | |
| Moments Australia (1) | | |

## 6.8 Hashtags

Hashtags were rarely utilized by Trump. Only 7 tweets out of 348 included a Hashtag. Two hashtag variations were used to refer to the coronavirus: #COVID19 and #COVID—19. The Coronavirus Aid, Relief, and Economic Security Act hashtag

#CARESAct appeared in two tweets while #MAGA which is a shortcut of Trump's 2016 campaign slogan Make America Great Again was used once. Although Trump used the nickname Do Nothing democrats very often in his tweets, the hashtag #DONOTHINGDEMOCRATS also appeared only once.

# 7 Discussion

"President Trump missed his chance to show that he could rise to the moment in the final chapter of his presidency and meet the defining challenge of his tenure", wrote a group of journalists in the New York Times nearly one year after the emergence of the coronavirus (SARS-CoV-2) in Wuhan China late December 2019 (Shear et al., 2020, December 31). Although arguably, there has been no other time during Trump's presidency, perhaps even the last decade, in which Americans looked for explanations and guidance from their President as much as during the COVID-19 pandemic. One that injected fear, uncertainty, and panic, into the lives of the entire world population. When citizens are deprived of certainty, they become "more inclined to take unsubstantiated propositions as facts, and opinions as knowledge" especially when coming from their leaders (Malouf, 2020, p. 1). Thus, even though presidential frames already poses a high degree of prominence arising from occupying the highest political office in the US and the ability to directly influence and shape "'facts on the ground'" (Entman, 2003, p. 422), crisis elevate the importance of the President's framing of issues, as citizens more than ever turn their heads to their leaders and rally in response to their handling and presentation of events (Baker & Oneal, 2001).

## 7.1 Denial

For this reason, this paper sought to explore what framing patterns dominated Trump's tweets about the COVID-19 Pandemic. The results show that from the early stages of the COVID-19 pandemic, Trump presented the public health crisis through a dominating political lens that downplayed the risk of the "situation" and failed to prepare the country and the public for upcoming stages and possible ramifications of a new airborne disease that does not differentiate between people based on their race, nationality or political affiliation, nor stop at borders (Trump, 2020, February 27a). Although the WHO declared the spread of COVID-19 a Public Health Emergency of International Concern in late January 2020 (see appendix), Trump's tweets throughout February to March 11, 2020, carried a framing pattern of denial and reassurance that fails to recognize the transnationality of the public health crisis. Despite indicating that "All countries working well together!", Trump's language differentiated between the risk COVID-19 poses on the US in comparison to other countries, drawing a binary picture in which the world is indeed facing a problem with "approximately 100,000 CoronaVirus cases worldwide, and 3,280 deaths" (Trump, 2020, February 27, March 5b) while China is undergoing a war to contain the virus. But, in the US the "Coronavirus is very much under control" and there is no need to worry about the possible severity of the disease, because his "quick" and "VERY EARLY" decision to close borders and "shut down" flights saved the country and kept the number of domestic infections and deaths low (Trump, 2020, February 28). Nonetheless, Trump didn't mention that the coronavirus was already spreading in the US when his decision took place. He also didn't explain that borders and flights were not "shut down", but merely restrictions for non-Americans coming from certain Chinese areas took place. At the same time, more than 27,000 Americans coming from mainland China entered the country within one month after the restrictions came into effect on February 2, 2020. Around 16,000 were lost track of and thus were not monitored by the government for possible infection with COVID-19 (Braun et al., 2020, July 18). But, perhaps Trump's clear distinction between who carried the virus into the country based on an insider vs. outsider categorization in a tweet published on March 5, 2020, in which Trump wrote that the US has "now, only 129 cases (40 Americans brought in) and 11 deaths" serves as an implicit moral justification of his decision (Trump, 2020, March 5b). One that reinforces fear from foreigners and identifies one homogenous group as "the pure people" in line with cultural populist beliefs by deflecting blame on the 'others' using an 'us' vs 'them' rhetoric (Mudde & Rovira Kaltwasser's, 2017, p. 6; Kyle & Meyer, 2020). "This is a virus that happened to pop up in China. But the virus doesn't discriminate between Asian versus non-Asian," said California Representative Ami Bera in a Congress hearing regarding the issue. Thus, choosing to differentiate between passengers based on their nationality, creates, "prejudices and harbor anxieties toward one population" (Ollstein, 2020, April 2). Bera's arguments come in congruence with the WHO's warning that, focusing on travel bans and restrictions as a solution for the spread of COVID-19 might "have the effect of increasing fear and stigma "(Shoichet, 2020, February 7). A phenomenon that has been continuously on the rise in many countries all over the world, especially in the US in which 3,795 discriminatory incidents against people of Asian descent were reported within only three months; March 2020 and February 2021 (Jeung et al., 2021, March 16; see chapter 2). Therefore, health experts' advice during such an early stage of the epidemic period was to mitigate border control policies arguing that "voluntary measures and education usually work better than edicts that may lead people to lie about their symptoms and travel history, and encourage countries to conceal outbreaks" (Ollstein, 2020, April 2; Turce, 2020, March 5). Dr. Jennifer Nuzzo, a senior scholar at the Johns Hopkins Center for Health Security, criticized February 5, 2020, Trump's decision to single out China for travel bans characterizing the move as a penalization for reporting cases. Especially, since respiratory viruses like the coronavirus "move quickly" and "are hard to spot because they look like many other diseases. It's very difficult to interrupt them at borders." The US "would need to have complete surveillance to do that" which it didn't have at the time. Therefore, the "virus could enter the U.S. from other parts of the world" (Farley, 2020, March 6). In that sense, WHO spokesperson Margaret Harris, advised governments that a lot of energy could be diverted when focusing on closing borders rather than protecting and equipping health workers, preparing health systems, and enhancing disease surveillance (Turce, 2020, March 5).

Nevertheless, Trump highlighted border closing and travel bans especially from China as the most suitable solution describing it as a "Godsend". Utilizing a religious metaphor that comes in close connection to the belief system of many Americans, could be interpreted as an attempt to elicit more resonance with his framing pattern. Keeping in mind that, culturally resonating elements help make a frame more "noticeable, understandable, memorable and emotionally charged" for the recipients (Entman, 2003, p. 417). On the other hand, vaccine development as a possible solution was only mentioned once in his tweets during the epidemic period (January 24 - March 10, 2020). However, it could be said that during this period, Trump's framing of China was, by far, more positive than in upcoming months with limited blaming messages. He portrayed

China as a cooperative and transparent country that is doing its best "to contain" the Coronavirus (Trump, 2020, January 24). Similarly, Trump maintained a positive and praiseful tone towards health professionals and governmental health agencies, reflecting a cooperative and functioning relationship with governmental health agencies during this period. But it gradually degraded with time to a point where the FDA was labeled as a "deep state" (Trump, 2020, August 22) during the second period ( March 11 - September 28, 2020) and a "slow turtle" (Trump, 2020, December 11) during the last period (November 4, 2020 - January 8, 2021).

However, the most alarming tweets within the Epidemic period were the ones in which Trump suggested that when the "weather starts to warm & the virus hopefully becomes weaker, and then gone" (Trump, 2020, February 7b) and compared the coronavirus to the seasonal Flu (Trump, 2020, March 9b). Thereby, making baseless evaluations that are not derived from science and failing to convey to the public the reality of uncertainty that surrounds the coronavirus. This reflects his main problem definition of the epidemic as a non-threatening situation that might end soon. According to Dr. Peter Hotez dean of the National School of Tropical Medicine at the Baylor College of Medicine, at the time Trump alleged that weather conditions could influence the coronavirus, a lot of things were still unknown about the nature of the virus to be able to make such assessments. Thus, it was "reckless" for the President to "assume that things will quiet down in spring and summer" (Kounang, 2020, February 7). Similarly, in a letter sent by members of the US National Academy of Sciences committee to the White House Office of Science and Technology Policy, the experts warned the Trump administration that: “Given that countries currently in ‘summer’ climates, such as Australia and Iran, are experiencing rapid virus spread, a decrease in cases with increases in humidity and temperature elsewhere should not be assumed.” (Relman, 2020, April 7). Moreover, studies raise a concern about the danger of comparing the death morality of the coronavirus to that of seasonal influenza, describing it as an “apples-to-oranges comparison” instead of “apples-to-apples comparison” (Faust & del Rio, 2020, p. 1046). In the US, mortality rates of the two diseases are obtained by the CDC through two completely different methods besides the fact that until mid-March the US COVID-19 testing capacity remained limited. In that sense, making direct comparisons between the two diseases disseminates “inaccurate information” and “threatens public health”. Thus, governmental officials who choose to draw such a comparison shows more concern about “re-open[ing] the economy and de-escalat[ing] mitigation strategies” than the public health (Faust & del Rio, 2020, p. 1046). Nonetheless, Trump didn’t drop equivalating between COVID-19 and seasonal influenza during the latter stages of the pandemic but rather explicitly continued to employ the contrast during the pre-election phase to campaign against lockdown measures in favor of reopening the economy as argued by Faust & del Rio (2020). Claiming on October 6, a day after his release from the hospital following his infection with the coronavirus that “Covid, in most populations”, is “far less lethal!!!” than the “Flu” (Trump, 2020, October 6a). The tweet came at a time in which the global COVID-19 death toll has surpassed one million with more than 210,000 deaths in the US in only eight months, which reflects the high degree of denial in Trump’s framing pattern of pandemic (see appendix). Later that day, it was flagged on

Twitter, citing that it "violated the Twitter Rules about spreading misleading and potentially harmful information related to COVID-19" (ABC News, 2020, October 6).

### 7.2 Downplaying the Threat

With the labeling of COVID-19 as a pandemic by the WHO on March 11, 2020 (Tedros Adhanom, 2020, March 11), war terminology started to appear more frequently in Trump's tweet in comparison to the epidemic period. However, in contrast to Benziman (2020) and Islentyeva (2020) who found Trump's official speeches about COVID-19 were dominated by war frames, it could be said that in his framing of COVID-19 on Twitter, Trump was not concerned with portraying the pandemic as a war, as much as, a "traditional security issue" as argued by Sondermann & Ulbert (2020, p. 315). Since security threats normally bring with them danger and fear, this line of framing allows leaders to propose "reactive emergency measures" rather than "long-term systemic approaches" and "transmits a sense of control" thereby shifting power to the executive and creating a cycle of securitizing the COVID-19 pandemic (Sondermann & Ulbert, 2020, p. 315). Between March 11 and September 28, 2020, Trump intensified his use of national security answers as the most suitable treatment recommendation, while mentioning public health measures such as social distancing only three times. Considering Bateson's (1972) argument that the inclusive function of frames automatically gives them an exclusive function as well; "Attend to what is within and do not attend to what is outside" (Bateson, 1972, p. 187). This further reflects the extent to which Trump failed to frame the COVID-19 as global public health, favoring the economy and the stock market. Nonetheless, not only did Trump exclude recommending public health measures, he actively framed them as being "worse" than the COVID-19 itself. On the contrary of health experts and scientific evidence about the role such public health measures play in slowing down the spread of the disease (Trump, 2020, March 24; Haberman & Sanger, 2020, March 23). As a result, Americans who have higher levels of faith in Trump were more likely to express willingness to disobey social distancing measures, break stay-at-home roles and go to social events (Graham et al., 2020). In Minnesota, protest organizers wearing Make America Great Again hats and waving Trump flags, adopted Trump's narrative in their Facebook invitation to protest against lockdown measures, reflecting a direct influence of his words: "Trump has been very clear that we must get America back to work very quickly or the 'cure' to this terrible disease may be the worse option!" (Hatemaker, 2020, April 17). Evidences, numbers and latest developments of science and scientific findings about the nature of the coronavirus, its threat, or possible health ramifications of COVID-19 were also excluded. This does not mean that Trump was entirely dismissive of scientific evidences. He was dismissive of scientific evidences and recommendations that didn't fit into his downplaying and economically focused framing pattern, or work in favor of his proposed solutions and appeals to the public. However, for example when prompting Hydrocholorquine, Trump citied a scientific study showing that the drug "cut the death rate significantly" (Trump, 2020, July 6b), which indicates that he was aware that using science as a source adds credibility to his argument and can be effective in shaping public opinion. At the same time, Trump didn't mention that experts warned him about the safety of the drug nor mentioned studies that questioned its effectiveness. A man died in the US while his wife was put in intensive care after drinking chloroquine phosphate, a substance used to treat fish. The wife said they were watching the President on TV talking about chloroquine before they took the substance (Associated Press, 2020, March 24). She said to the press: "Trump kept saying it was basically pretty much a cure" (Associated Press, 2020, March 24).

### 7.3 The Chinese Virus

Another dangerous framing pattern offered by Trump was activated on March 16, 2020, with the help of a single rhetorical framing device; the "Chinese Virus". He wrote: "The United States will be powerfully supporting those industries, like Airlines and others, that are particularly affected by the Chinese Virus. We will be stronger than ever before!" (Trump, 2020, March 16). In light of the power, Trump presides over, given his control over the government apparatus and the hybridity of the current media system (Chadwick, 2017; Entman, 2003), his use of an ethnically-focused framing device was carried out simultaneously and intersectionality throughout the different levels of the cascading activation model, as the term occupied news headlines of all types of media outlets as well as debates on social media platforms (Entman, 2003; Entman & Usher, 2018;). However, this is not to say that the term "Chinese virus" by itself is the only component that built up Trump's main framing pattern of COVID-19 during the pandemic period, but could rather be viewed as a linguistic vehicle that carried it out (Entman, 1993, p. 52). Thereby, reflecting Laktoff's (2014, p. 2) argument that framing "is about getting language that fits your worldview. It is not just language. The ideas are primary—and the language carries those ideas, evokes those ideas." With his naming of the COVID-19 Trump as the "Chinese virus", "China virus" and "Chinese plague" brought terms that fit right into his worldview and used them to define the public health crisis. A cultural populist worldview that distinguishes between 'us' and 'them' and amplifies anti-immigrant rhetoric and xenophobia. According to Malouf (2020, p. 3) using the "Chinese virus" implicitly suggests that: (1) "Chinese people are responsible for the origination and spread of the virus, (2)" Chinese people are more likely to be carriers of the virus.", (3) "Individuals of Chinese origin are distinct from American citizens." (Malouf, 2020, p. 3). Thus, the term is especially dangerous considering that its ambiguity allows speakers to easily refute such propositions when criticized while giving listeners the room to interpret the term as they wish (Malouf, 2020). As a result, terms like the "China virus" and the "Chinese virus" were explicitly used in attacks against people of Asian descent which have been on the rise in countries all over the world, especially in the US (see chapter 2). Nonetheless, Trump was more concerned with deflecting blame on China than protecting the Asian community. Thus, in line with Altheide (2020, 529) this paper finds that coming up with a name that connects China and the Chinese people to the coronavirus was part of Trump's "blame game", which included blaming China, blaming the media, blaming the Obama administration, blaming Democrats and the Democratic party as well as blaming scientists and other political actors who criticize him (see also, Yamey & Gonsalves, 2020; Rutledge, 2020). Even the World Health Organization was blamed by Trump for the spread of the coronavirus and described as too slow in its response in an attempt to deflect attention from his delayed response. "President Trump attacked others and promoted border closings to counter his vulnerability for denying the threat of the virus on the United States" (Altheide, 2020, p. 530). When Trump sought to mitigate the effects of his xenophobic rhetoric on people of Asian descent saying that "the spreading of the Virus is NOT their fault in any way, shape, or form", he still failed to distance himself from the language that activates the neural-circuits of the blame frame (Lakoff, 2014; see chapter 3.5.2).

## 7.4 Blame Game

Both the media and Democrats were main targets of Trump's blaming messages during the Pandemic period. They were accused of exaggerating the threat and politicizing the COVID-19 pandemic to undermine his successful handling of the COVID-19 pandemic. This was done with the help of insult, mocking, and naming politics as well as the Twitter mention function to single out enemies and identify blame targets. This speaks to Lakoff's (2016, July 23) argument that Trump's communication style operates following the motto: "Naming is Identifying" (Lakoff 2016, July 23; see chapter 4.1.3). Trump also tried to draw a picture of the US media and Democrats as being more on China's side than their own country because they fail to blame the spread of COVID-19 on China. Indicating that, Democrats were seeking to benefit from their "their cash cow" country (Trump, 2020, May 2). While for example, The "Fake News" New York Times was "recently thrown out of China like dogs, and obviously, want back in." (Trump, 2020, April 11). Trump also, employed the Swine Flu pandemic as a tool to further attack and denounce Democrats and the Obama Administration, especially his 2020 election rival Joe Biden. Accusing them of failing to handle the H1N1 pandemic in 2009 while praising himself and his administration for doing a much better job. Although, COVID-19 is by far, deadlier than the Swine Flu pandemic (CDC, 2019, June 11; Adhanom Ghebreyesus, 2020, April 13). Thereby, again, downplaying the threat of COVID-19 and turning it into a political weapon to campaign for his re-election in November 2020. As put by journalist Philip Bump (2020, May 26):

> Likely, he generally thinks he is merely nudging outward the boundaries of reality even when he's far outside them. But he knows that he can simply push an idea out into the world and watch his supporters and defenders attach themselves to it, working to build up pearls from any grain of sand.

### 7.5 Pandemic Politics

This line of politicalizing the Pandemic was intensified with the start of the first election debate on 29, September 2020. Tweets were centered around drawing a rosy picture of reality and the US economy. In full ignorance of the human death toll and consequences of the COVID-19 pandemic. Even after his infection with COVID-19, he focused on reflecting strength, thereby minimizing the effects of the coronavirus and defining it as being non-threatening. While at the same not letting this opportunity pass him by without using it to practice praise for himself and his Administration: "Don't be afraid of Covid. Don't let it dominate your life. We have developed, under the Trump Administration, some great drugs & knowledge. I feel better than I did 20 years ago!", he said (Trump, 2020, October 5b). His tweet elicited anger and frustration among COVID-19 survivors and families of victims, who found the President remarks to be highly inconsiderate and dangerous, raising awareness that there is no chance not to let COVID-19 dominate your life when it deprives you of your health and takes away loved ones (Medaris Miller, 2020, October 6). Especially, since at the time Trump was receiving "top-of-the-line" health care and treatments, average Americans were struggling to even be able to get tested, hospitals were reaching full capacity and running short on ventilators thereby hasting the deaths of thousands (Wong, 2020, October 8). However, the dangerous effect of the Trump framing pattern can be reflected by the fact that some families reported that their fellow members of the community refused to accept COVID-19 as the reason behind the death of loved ones (Abrams, 2020, November 19). Similarly, many medical staff members reported receiving COVID-19 patients who refused to acknowledge their infection with the disease, because it simply doesn't exist (Falzone, 2020, November 19). A nurse working in the COVID-19 area of a Californian hospital was even mocked by a patient for wearing a mask to protect herself. "What's the matter, are you a Democrat or something?", he said. While the nurse asserted that: "Every single person I have encountered who was misinformed on COVID-19 referenced the president's dishonesty on Fox News or social media" (Falzone, 2020, November 19). According to the Pew Research center (Schaeffer, 2020, July 24), a quarter of US adults see at least some truth in COVID-19 conspiracy theories, with Republicans (34%) being more inclined to do so than Democrats (18%). This is not surprising considering that a "key strain of the president's narrative is that concerns about the coronavirus are being weaponized by bad-faith actors—a notion that has spawned a broad range of conspiracy theories", as put by journalist McKay Coppins (2020, March 11).

The results of this paper reflect Coppins's assertion. Trump, indeed, weaponized the COVID-19 Pandemic as a method to attack Biden by focusing on the economic drawbacks of lockdown policies rather than the public health issues. These attempts to portray members of the US political and medical elite as "bad-faith actors" parallels populist ideologies in "identifying 'folk devils' and creating moral panics, whereby apparent threats to collective interests are amplified through inflammatory rhetoric" (Mannion & Speed, 2020, p. 7). Hence, he employed populism as a communication style, focusing on dramatization and the "need to generate tension in order to build up support [...] by denouncing the tragedies that would befall the community if it were to be deprived of its defences" (Albertazzi, 2007 p. 335). While at the same time practicing extensive self-praise, which was the main reason behind deploying quotes as technical framing devices. Almost all quotes used by Trump originated from conservative voices, especially Fox News shows and media personas thereby widening the "Fox-Trump feedback loop" (Altheide, 2020, p. 524). The quotes were either complimentary of his response, or critical of his opponents, in line with Benziman (2020) findings. After election day on November 4, 2020, self-praising and crediting himself for the development of the vaccines was the main focus of Trump's tweets, besides issuing attacks on the media, Joe Biden, and the FDA. Trump aimed to ensure that he only gets the credit for the development of the vaccines; For those great "historians", please remember that these great discoveries, which will end the China Plague, all took place on my watch!" (Trump, 2020, November 16). Meanwhile, science and health institutions especially the FDA, were given no credit at all but instead undermined, insulted, and accused of politicizing the vaccine approval process.

This study provides empirical evidence on how Trump used Twitter to politicalize the pandemic. Showing that he was more concerned with practicing pandemic politics, issuing attacks on science and scientists thereby jeopardizing the public's response to health measures than acknowledging their role in mitigating the effects of the pandemic. Trump spoke "force, aggression, anger, and no shame" issuing attacks on China, the media, the Democratic Party, scientists, and governmental health institutions and weaponizing public health measures such as lockdowns to evoke anger towards the political elite and his opponents (Lakoff, 2016). While at the same time using non-threatening and reassuring language to downplay the threat of the COVID-19 pandemic and prioritize the economy over the public health. Considering the extensive media attention given to Trump's framing pattern during the COVID-19 pandemic and the above-mentioned developments it elicited.

## 7.6 Limitations and Future Work

The results of this study could be used by educationalists and journalists to explicitly illustrate how Twitter was utilized by Trump to continuously shape and reshape public opinion, media headlines, and social media discussions and turn a public health crisis into a political one (Altheide, 2020). Thereby, offering a modern-day reflection of Entman's (2003, p. 417) definition of framing as "the central process by which government officials and journalists exercise political power over each other and the public".

However, this study also has its limitations; It excluded retweets, focusing only on analyzing Trump's original tweets. Thus, it would be useful for further studies to build up upon the its findings by comparing them to framing patterns of the COVID-19 pandemic in Trump's retweets. Especially, considering that this study failed to offer detailed insight into the types of hyperlinks Trump relied on for two reasons; First, most embedded hyperlinks redirected back to his suspended account. Second, analyzing the content of the links fell out of the scope of the paper. Thus, analyzing retweets as well as the type of content embedded in Trump's original tweets can bring more useful insights about Trump's framing patterns and the type of sources and information he relied on. As well as the voices he chose to amplify via his Twitter account during the COVID-19 pandemic. Moreover, although this study tried to explain tweets within their context, explicitly fact-checking the information provided in Trump's tweets could better help scholars in understanding how much of Trump's framing of the COVID-19 pandemic was carried out with the help of false information. Lastly, this paper was focused on understanding how meaning is constructed through framing messages on the communicators' side, therefore future studies that explore the effect of Trump's framing patterns on recipients' will be very complementary to this study.

## 8 References

Abbas, A. H. (2019). Super-Hyperbolic Man: Hyperbole as an Ideological Discourse Strategy in Trump's Speeches. *International Journal for the Semiotics of Law-Revue internationale de Sémiotique juridique*, 32(2), 505-522.

ABC News (2020, October 6). *Twitter, Facebook flag Donald Trump comparing COVID-19 to the flu.* ABC News. https://www.abc.net.au/news/2020-10-07/donald-trump-covid19-coronavirus-twitter-facebook/12737660

Abrams, A. (2020, November 19). *'My Frustration Turned Into Anger.' Some Americans Who Lost Family Members to COVID-19 Have Turned Against Donald Trump.* Time. https://time.com/5913055/covid-19-grief-politics-trump/

Adhanom Ghebreyesus, T. (2020, December 27). *International Day of Epidemic Preparedness*. [Video]. Youtube. https://www.youtube.com/watch?v=sMnhWcptYp8&feature=emb_title

Adhanom Ghebreyesus, T. (2020, April 4). *WHO says Covid-19 is 10 times more deadly than swine flu.* France 24. https://www.france24.com/en/20200413-who-says-covid-19-is-10-times-more-deadly-than-swine-flu

Adolph, C., Amano, K., Bang-Jensen, B., Fullman, N., & Wilkerson, J. (2020). Pandemic politics: Timing state-level social distancing responses to COVID-19. *Journal of Health Politics, Policy and Law*, 46 (2), 211-233.

Al-Azzawi, Q. O. & Hameed, R. K. (2020). The pragmatics of hyperbole in Trump's presidential speeches concerning coronavirus crisis. *Journal of Critical Reviews*, 7(13), 2394-5125.

Albertazzi, D. (2007). Addressing 'the People': A Comparative Study of the Lega Nord's and Lega dei Ticinesi's Political Rhetoric and Styles of Propaganda. *Modern Italy*, 12(3), 327-347.

Albertazzi, D., & McDonnell, D. (2008). *Twenty-first century populism: The spectre of Western European democracy*. Palgrave Macmillan.

AllSides (2021). *AllSides Media Bias Chart.* AllSides. https://www.allsides.com/media-bias/media-bias-chart

Alter, S. M., Maki, D. G., LeBlang, S., Shih, R. D., & Hennekens, C. H. (2020). The menacing assaults on science, FDA, CDC, and health of the US public. EClinicalMedicine, 27.

American Journal of Managed Care (2020, Januaury 1). *A Timeline of COVID-19 Developments in 2020.* https://www.ajmc.com/view/a-timeline-of-covid19-developments-in-2020

Annas, G. (1995). Reframing the debate on health care reform by replacing our metaphors. *New England Journal of Medicine*, 332(11), 744–747.

Altheide, D. L. (2020). Pandemic in the Time of Trump: Digital Media Logic and Deadly Politics. *Symbolic Interaction*, 43(3), 514-540.

Alvarado, A. (2020, June 20). *Trump: Fauci has nothing to do with football.* Live 5 WCSC. https://www.live5news.com/2020/06/20/trump-fauci-has-nothing-do-with-football/

Aral, S. (2020, November 2*). Revealed: Joe Biden has been hit harder by Twitter's new retweet policy than Donald Trump.* NewStatesman https://www.newstatesman.com/world/2020/11/revealed-joe-biden-has-been-hit-harder-twitter-s-new-retweet-policy-donald-trump

Ariely, G. (2016). Why does patriotism prevail? Contextual explanations of patriotism across countries. *Identities*, 24, 1–27.

Aronsson, K. (2002). Goffman, vetandet och den allvarsamma leken [Goffman, knowing andserious play]. In P. Linell & K. Aronsson (Eds.), Jagen och resterna: Goffman, Viveka ochsamtalet (pp. 63â74).

Aslam, S. (2018). *Twitter by the numbers: Stats, demographics & fun facts*. Omnicoreagency. Com.https://www.omnicoreagency.com/twitter-statistics/#:~:text=Twitter%20Demographics,(users%20outside%20the%20U.S.)

Associated Press (2020, March 24). *Arizona man dies after attempting to take Trump coronavirus'cure"cure'*. The Guardian. https://www.theguardian.com/world/2020/mar/24/coronavirus-cure-kills-man-after-trump-touts-chloroquine-phosphate

Avlon, J. (2021, March 18). *Why anti-Asian American violence is rising -- along with White supremacist propaganda*. CNN. https://edition.cnn.com/2021/03/17/opinions/asian-hate-crimes-us-avlon/index.html

Baker, W. D., & Oneal, J. R. (2001). Patriotism or opinion leadership: The nature and origins of the "rally 'round the flag" effect. *The Journal of Conflict Resolution*, 45, 661–687.

Bar Tal, D., & Staub, E. (Eds.). (1997). *Patriotism in the lives of individuals and nations*. Nelson-Hall Publishers.

Bar-Tal, D. (2013). *Ethos of conflict*. Cambridge University Press.

Barro, R. J., Ursúa, J. F., & Weng, J. (2020). *The coronavirus and the great influenza pandemic: Lessons from the "spanish flu" for the coronavirus's potential effects on mortality and economic activity* (No. w26866). National Bureau of Economic Research.

Bateson, G. (1956). *The message 'This is play'*. In B. Schaffner (Ed.), Group processes: Transactions of the second conference (pp. 145–242). Josiah Macy Jr. Foundation.

Bateson, G. (1972). A theory of play and fantasy. *Psychiatric Research Reports*, 2, 39-5.

BBC (2020, January 14). *Trump impeached for 'inciting' US Capitol riot in historic second charge*. BBC News. https://www.bbc.com/news/world-us-canada-55656385

Bennett, W. L. (1990). Toward a theory of press state relations in the United States. *Journal of communication*, 40(2), 103-127.

Bennett, W. L., & Serrin, W. (2005). *The watchdog role. The press*, 169, 188.

Benziman, Y. (2020). “Winning” the “battle” and “beating” the COVID-19 “enemy”: Leaders’ use of war frames to define the pandemic. Peace and Conflict: *Journal of Peace Psychology*, 26(3), 247.

Berzleja, Z., & Kertész, F. (2020). Donald Trump’s Communication During COVID-19 Pandemic On Twitter. http://ls00012.mah.se/handle/2043/32833

Biden, J. (2021, January 26). *Memorandum Condemning and Combating Racism, Xenophobia, and Intolerance Against Asian Americans and Pacific Islanders in the United States*. The White House. https://www.whitehouse.gov/briefing-room/presidential-actions/2021/01/26/memorandum-condemning-and-combating-racism-xenophobia-and-intolerance-against-asian-americans-and-pacific-islanders-in-the-united-states/

Biden, J. (2021, January 6). *Biden calls on Trump to go on national TV and demand end to 'siege' on Capitol*. Fox 2 Detroit. https://www.fox2detroit.com/news/president-elect-joe-biden-to-speak-as-chaos-erupts-at-us-capitol

Block, E., & Negrine, R. (2017). The populist communication style: Toward a critical framework. *International Journal of Communication Systems*, 11, 178-197.

Blok, A. (2001). *Honour and violence*. Polity Press.

Bolsen, T., Palm, R., & Kingsland, J. T. (2020). <? covid19?> Framing the Origins of COVID-19. *Science Communication*, 42(5), 562-585.

Bolsonaro, J. (2020, March 23). *Brazil's Jair Bolsonaro says coronavirus crisis is a media trick*. The Guardian. https://www.theguardian.com/world/2020/mar/23/brazils-jair-bolsonaro-says-coronavirus-crisis-is-a-media-trick

Boot, M. (2020, May 6). *Opinion: Trump isn’t the only populist leader losing the battle against the coronavirus*. Washington Post.

https://www.washingtonpost.com/opinions/2020/05/06/trump-isnt-only-populist-leader-losing-battle-against-coronavirus/

Borah, P. (2011). Conceptual issues in framing theory: A systematic examination of a decade's literature. *Journal of communication*, 61(2), 246-263.

Borah, P. (2020). *Trump's poor relationship with the media has made the US Covid-19 outbreak worse*. USApp-American Politics and Policy Blog. http://eprints.lse.ac.uk/104376/1/Borah_trumps_poor_relationship_with_the_media_has_made_the_us_covid_outbreak.pdf

Bos, L., Van der Brug, W., & De Vreese, C. (2011). How the media shape perceptions of right-wing populist leaders. *Political Communication*, 28(2), 182-206.

Boydstun, A. E., Gross, J. H., Resnik, P., & Smith, N. A. (2013, September). *Identifying media frames and frame dynamics within and across policy issues*. In New Directions in Analyzing Text as Data Workshop, London.

Braun, S., Yen, H. & Woodward, C. AP FACT CHECK: *Trump and the virus-era China ban that isn't*. AP News. https://apnews.com/article/d227b34b168e576bf5068b92a03c003d

Bucy, E. P., Foley, J. M., Lukito, J., Doroshenko, L., Shah, D. V., Pevehouse, J. C., & Wells, C. (2020). performing populism: trump's transgressive debate style and the dynamics of Twitter response. *New Media & Society*, 22(4), 634-658.

Bump, P. (2020, May 26). Trump's comparison of the coronavirus to H1N1 in 2009 distills to 'but Obama'. The Washington Post. https://www.washingtonpost.com/politics/2020/05/26/trumps-comparison-coronavirus-h1n1-2009-distills-obama/

Byers, D. (2017, February 22). *Media more trustworthy than Trump, poll finds*. CNN. http://money.cnn.com/2017/02/22/media/trump-media-trustquinnipiac/?mc_cid=2fc95ae03c&mc_eid=b89abdbf0b

Byler,. D (2020, October 6). *This is Trump's worst tweet ever. No, really. Washington post.* https://www.washingtonpost.com/opinions/2020/10/06/this-is-trumps-worst-tweet-ever-no-really/

Cacciatore, M. A., Scheufele, D. A., & Iyengar, S. (2016). The end of framing as we know it… and the future of media effects. *Mass Communication and Society*, 19(1), 7-23.

Callaghan, K., & Schnell, F. (2000). Media frames, public attitudes, and elite response: An analysis of the gun control issue. *Public Integrity*, 1, 343–358.

Carretón Ballester, M. C., & López Villafranca, P. (2016). The impact of the Ebola Virus and rare diseases in the media and the perception of risk in Spain. *Catalan Journal of Communication & Cultural Studies*, 8(2), 245-263.

Center for the Study of Hate and Extremism [CSUSB] (2021, March 2). *Fact Sheet: Anti-Asian Prejudice 2020*. CSUSB. https://www.csusb.edu/sites/default/files/FACT%20SHEET-%20Anti-Asian%20Hate%202020%203.2.21.pdf

Centers for Disease Control and Prevention [CDC] (2020, January 21). *First Travel-related Case of 2019 Novel Coronavirus Detected in United States*. CDC. https://www.cdc.gov/media/releases/2020/p0121-novel-coronavirus-travel-case.html

Centre for Disease Control and Prevention (2012). Lesson 1: Introduction to Epidemiology. CDC. https://www.cdc.gov/csels/dsepd/ss1978/lesson1/section11.html

Chadwick, A. (2017). *The hybrid media system: Politics and power*. Oxford University Press.

Chang, C., Lee, A. & Othagaki, J. (2021, March 12). *Anti-Asian Attacks Are Blighting the United States*. Foreign Policy. https://foreignpolicy.com/2021/03/12/anti-asian-attacks-united-states-covid/

Chong, D., & Druckman, J. N. (2007a). Framing theory. *Annu. Rev. Polit. Sci.*, 10, 103-126.

Chong, D., & Druckman, J. N. (2007b). A theory of framing and opinion formation in competitive elite environments. *Journal of communication*, 57(1), 99-118.

Christodoulidou, M. (2011). Hyperbole in everyday conversation. *Selected papers on theoretical and applied linguistics*, 19, 143-152.

Cinelli, M., Quattrociocchi, W., Galeazzi, A., Valensise, C. M., Brugnoli, E., Schmidt, A. L., ... & Scala, A. (2020). The covid-19 social media infodemic. arXiv preprint arXiv:2003.05004.

Claridge, C. (2011). *Hyperbole in English: A corpus-based study of exaggeration.* Cambridge University Press.

Colleoni, E., Rozza, A., & Arvidsson, A. (2014). Echo chamber or public sphere? Predicting political orientation and measuring political homophily in Twitter using big data. *Journal of communication*, 64(2), 317-332.

Collinson, S. (2020). *Trump closes his campaign by insulting Fauci for telling the truth.* CNN. https://edition.cnn.com/2020/10/20/politics/donald-trump-anthony-fauci-coronavirus/index.html

Connolly-Ahern, C. & Broadway, S.C. (2008). "To Booze or No to Booze?" Newspaper Coverage of Foetal Alcohol Spectrum Disorders. Science Communication, 29 (3), 366-370.

Cooper, M. (2016, September, 27). *Donald Trump's great, tremendous, unbelievable penchant for hyperbole at the first presidential debate*. Quartz. https://qz.com/792825/presidential-debate-donald-trumps-great-tremendous-unbelievable-penchant-for-hyperbole/

Coppins, M. (2020, March 11). *Trump's Dangerously Effective Coronavirus Propaganda: The President's Effort to Play Down the Pandemic Is Being Amplified by a Coalition of Partisan Media, Digital Propagandists, and White House Officials*. The Atlantic. https://www.theatlantic.com/politics/archive/2020/03/trump-coronavirus-threat/607825/

Council on American-Islamic Relations [CAIR] (n.d). *IN: Meaning of 'Jihad' Misunderstood by Many*. CAIR. https://www.cair.com/cair_in_the_news/in-meaning-of-jihad-misunderstood-by-many/

Crayne, M. P., & Medeiros, K. E. (2020). Making sense of crisis: Charismatic, ideological, and pragmatic leadership in response to COVID-19. *American Psychologist*. Advance online publication. https://doi.org/10.1037/amp0000715

D'Angelo, P. (2019). Beyond Framing: A Forum for Framing Researchers. In: D'Angelo, P., Lule, J., Neuman, W. R., Rodriguez, L., Dimitrova, D. V., & Carragee, K. M. (2019). Beyond framing: A forum for framing researchers. *Journalism & mass communication quarterly*, 96(1), 12-30.

D'ANGELO, P. A. U. L., & Kuypers, J. A. (2010). Introduction: Doing news framing analysis. In Doing news framing analysis (pp. 17-30). Routledge.

D'Angelo, P., Lule, J., Neuman, W. R., Rodriguez, L., Dimitrova, D. V., & Carragee, K. M. (2019). Beyond framing: A forum for framing researchers. *Journalism & mass communication quarterly*, 96(1), 12-30.

Dan, V., & Raupp, J. (2018). A systematic review of frames in news reporting of health risks: Characteristics, construct consistency vs. name diversity, and the relationship of frames to framing functions. *Health, Risk & Society*, 20(5-6), 203-226.

Darcy, O. (2019). *How Twitter's algorithm is amplifying extreme political rhetoric*. CNN Business. https://edition.cnn.com/2019/03/22/tech/twitter-algorithm-political-rhetoric/index.html

Dastgeer, S., & Onyebadi, U. (2020). Presidential Communication in the "Tweetosphere": A Functional and Network Analyses of President Trump's Direct Messaging. *The Journal of Social Media in Society*, 9(1), 156-179.

David, C. C., Atun, J. M., Fille, E., & Monterola, C. (2011). Finding frames: Comparing two methods of frame analysis. *Communication Methods and Measures*, 5(4), 329-351.

Dawsey (2018, January 12). *Trump derides protections for immigrants from 'shithole' countries*. Washington Post. https://www.washingtonpost.com/politics/trump-attacks-protections-for-immigrants-from-shithole-countries-in-oval-office-meeting/2018/01/11/bfc0725c-f711-11e7-91af-31ac729add94_story.html

De Vreese, C. H. (2012). New avenues for framing research. *American behavioral scientist*, 56(3), 365-375.

De Vreese, C. H., & Lecheler, S. (2012). News framing research: An overview and new developments. The SAGE handbook of political communication, 292-306.

De Vreese, C. H., Esser, F., Aalberg, T., Reinemann, C., & Stanyer, J. (2018). Populism as an expression of political communication content and style: A new perspective. *The international journal of press/politics*, 23(4), 423-438.

Deetz, S. A., Tracy, S. J., & Simpson, J. L. (1999). *Leading organizations through transition: Communication and cultural change*. Sage Publications.

Denk, H. (2011). *Twitter and Political Communication: Conceptualization and Empirical Findings* (Vol. 307). GRIN Verlag.

Deslatte, A. (2020). To shop or shelter? Issue framing effects and social-distancing preferences in the COVID-19 pandemic. *Journal of Behavioral Public Administration*, 3(1).

Detsky, A. S., & Bogoch, I. I. (2020). COVID-19 in Canada: Experience and response. *Jama*, 324(8), 743-744.

Donald, J. Trump for President. (2016, January 28). *Political correctness* [Video]. Youtube.https://www.youtube.com/watch?v=SYIinBKejnM&index=7&list=PLKOAoICmbyV3Q7PLQnzDfpqzXrCWRTTE8

Dredge, S. (2014). *Yes, Twitter is putting tweets in your timeline from people you don't follow*. The Guardian. https://www.theguardian.com/technology/2014/oct/17/twitter-tweets-timeline-dont-follow

Drylie-Carey, L., Sánchez-Castillo, S., & Galán-Cubillo, E. (2020). European leaders unmasked: Covid-19 communication strategy through Twitter. *El Profesional de la Información*, 29(5).

Dunning, E. (2018). # trumpstyle: the political frames and Twitter attacks of Donald Trump. *The Journal of Social Media in Society*, 7(2), 205-231.

effects in a two-wave panel study. Studies in Communication Sciences, 8(2), 101-128.

Elo, S., & Kyngäs, H. (2008). The qualitative content analysis process. *Journal of advanced nursing*, 62(1), 107-115.

Engel Bromwich, J. (2016). *What Is Breitbart News?*. The New York Times. https://www.nytimes.com/2016/08/18/business/media/what-is-breitbart-news.html

Engesser, S., Fawzi, N., & Larsson, A. O. (2017). Populist online communication: Introduction to the special issue. *Information, Communication & Society*, 20 (9), 1279-1292.

Enli, G. (2017). Twitter as arena for the authentic outsider: exploring the social media campaigns of Trump and Clinton in the 2016 US presidential election. *European journal of communication*, 32(1), 50-61.

Entman, R. M. (1993). Framing: Toward Clarification of a Fractured Paradigm. *Journal of Communication*, 43(4), 51-58.

Entman, R. M. (2003). Cascading activation: Contesting the White House's frame after 9/11. *Political Communication*, 20(4), 415-432.

Entman, R. M. (2004). *Projections of power: Framing news, public opinion, and US foreign policy*. University of Chicago Press.

Entman, R. M. (2007). Framing bias: Media in the distribution of power. *Journal of communication*, 57(1), 163-173.

Entman, R. M., & Usher, N. (2018). Framing in a fractured democracy: Impacts of digital technology on ideology, power and cascading network activation. *Journal of Communication*, 68(2), 298-308.

Epstein, J. (1992). AIDS, stigma and narratives of containment. American Imago, 49(3), 293–310. *European Journal of Interactive Multimedia and Education*, 1(2), e02006.

Evanega, S., Lynas, M., Adams, J., Smolenyak, K., & Insights, C. G. (2020). Coronavirus misinformation: quantifying sources and themes in the COVID-19 'infodemic'. *JMIR Preprints*.

Eysenbach, G. (2020). How to fight an infodemic: The four pillars of infodemic management. *Journal of medical Internet research*, 22(6), e21820.

Fairhurst, G. & Sarr, R. (1996). *The art of Framing*. San Francisco: Jossey-Bass.

Fairhurst, G. T. (2005). Reframing the art of framing: Problems and prospects for leadership. *Leadership*, 1(2), 165-185.

Falzone, D. (2020, November 19). *"It's the Trump Bubble": The Right Has Created a Wave of COVID Patients Who Don't Believe It's Real.* Vanity Fair. https://www.vanityfair.com/news/2020/11/a-wave-of-covid-patients-who-dont-believe-its-real

Farely, R. (2020, March 6). *The Facts on Trump's Travel Restrictions*. FactCheck.org. https://www.factcheck.org/2020/03/the-facts-on-trumps-travel-restrictions/

Fauci, A. (2020, December 9). *When Public Health Means Business. Harvard T.H. Chan School of Public Health.* https://www.hsph.harvard.edu/coronavirus/covid-19-news-and-resources/when-public-health-means-business/

Faust, J. S., & Del Rio, C. (2020). Assessment of deaths from COVID-19 and from seasonal influenza. *JAMA internal medicine*, 180(8), 1045-1046.

Federal Bureau of Investigation [FBI] (n.d.). *Hate Crimes*. FBI. https://www.fbi.gov/investigate/civil-rights/hate-crimes

Festinger, L. (1957). *A theory of cognitive dissonance* (Vol. 2). Stanford university press.

Fisher, H. (2008). *Self, logic, and figurative thinking*. Columbia University Press.

Goffman, E. (1974). F*rame analysis: An essay on the organization of experience*. Harvard University Press.

Flynn, D. J., Nyhan, B., & Reifler, J. (2017). The nature and origins of misperceptions: Understanding false and unsupported beliefs about politics. *Political Psychology*, 38, 127-150.

Foley, K., Ward, P., & McNaughton, D. (2019). Innovating qualitative framing analysis for purposes of media analysis within public health inquiry. *Qualitative Health Research*, 29(12), 1810-1822.

Forgey, Q. (2020, March 18). *Trump on 'Chinese virus' label: 'It's not racist at all'. Politico*. https://www.politico.com/news/2020/03/18/trump-pandemic-drumbeat-coronavirus-135392

Fourie, P. J. (Ed.). (2001). Media Studies: Institutions, theories, and issues (Vol. 1). Juta and Company Ltd.

Fujiwara, T., Müller, K., & Schwarz, C. (2020). *How Twitter affected the 2016 presidential election*. VoxEU. https://voxeu.org/article/how-twitter-affected-2016-presidential-election

Funk, C., Kennedy, B., & Johnson, C. [Pew Research Center] (2020). *Science and scientists held in high esteem across global publics*. Pew Research Center. https://www.pewresearch.org/science/2020/09/29/science-and-scientists-held-in-high-esteem-across-global-publics/

Gadde, V. & Beykpour, K. (2020, November 12).An *update on our work around the 2020 US Elections*. Twitter. https://blog.twitter.com/en_us/topics/company/2020/2020-election-update.html

Gadde, V. & Beykpour, K. (2020, October 9). *Additional steps we're taking ahead of the 2020 US Election*. Twitter. https://blog.twitter.com/official/en_us/topics/company/2020/2020-election-changes.html

Gallagher, J. (2020). *Dexamethasone, Remdesivir, Regeneron: Trump's Covid treatment explained.* BBC. https://www.bbc.com/news/health-54418464

Gambino, L. (2021, January 9). *Trump has lost Twitter, his biggest political megaphone. Now what?*.The Guardian. https://www.theguardian.com/us-news/2021/jan/08/trump-has-lost-twitter-his-biggest-political-megaphone-now-what

Gamson, W. A. & Modigliani, A. (1989). Media discourse and public opinion on nuclear: A constructionist approach. *American Journal of Sociology*, 95, 1-37.

Gitlin, T. (1980). *The whole world is watching: Mass media in the making and unmaking of the making and unmaking of the new left*. Berkeley, CA: University of California Press.

Giuffrida, A., & Willsher, K. (2020). *Outbreaks of xenophobia in west as coronavirus spreads*. The Guardian. https://www.theguardian.com/world/2020/jan/31/spate-of-anti-chinese-incidents-in-italy-amid-coronavirus-panic

Golbeck, J., Grimes, J. M., & Rogers, A. (2010). Twitter use by the US Congress. *Journal of the American Society for Information Science and Technology*, 61(8), 1612-1621.

Google Trends (2020). *See what was trending in 2020*. Google. https://trends.google.com/trends/yis/2020/GLOBAL/

Graham, A., Cullen, F. T., Pickett, J. T., Jonson, C. L., Haner, M., & Sloan, M. M. (2020). Faith in Trump, moral foundations, and social distancing Defiance during the coronavirus pandemic. *Socius*, 6, 1-23.

Grant, J. A., & Hundley, H. (2009). Images of the war on cancer in the Associated Press: centering survivors and marginalizing victims. *American Communication Journal*, 11(4), 1-16.

Haberman, M. (2020, April 20). *Trump, Head of Government, Leans Into Antigovernment Message*. The New York Times. https://www.nytimes.com/2020/04/20/us/politics/trump-coronavirus.html

Haberman, M & Sanger, D. E. (2020, March 23). rump Says Coronavirus Cure Cannot 'Be Worse Than the Problem Itself'. The New York Times. https://www.nytimes.com/2020/03/23/us/politics/trump-coronavirus-restrictions.html

Hallahan, K. (1999). Seven models of framing: Implications for public relations. *Journal of public relations research*, 11(3), 205-242.

Halliday, M.A.K. & Hasan.R.(1976). *Cohesion in English*. Longman Group Limited.

Haman, M. (2020). The use of Twitter by state leaders and its impact on the public during the COVID-19 pandemic. *Heliyon*, 6(11), e05540.

Hart, P. S., Chinn, S., & Soroka, S. (2020). <? covid19?> Politicization and Polarization in COVID-19 News Coverage. *Science Communication*, 42(5), 679-697.

Hatemaker, T. (2020, April 17). *Trump's hype for state lockdown protests puts Twitter and Facebook's new COVID-19 policies to the test*. Tech Crunch. https://techcrunch.com/2020/04/17/coronavirus-protests-trump-liberate-minnesota-tweets-facebook-twitter/

Hemphill, L., Culotta, A., & Heston, M. (2013). Framing in Social Media: How the US Congress uses Twitter hashtags to frame political issues. Available at SSRN 2317335.

Hertog, J. K., & McLeod, D. M. (2001). *A multiperspectival approach to framing analysis: A field guide. Framing public life: Perspectives on media and our understanding of the social world,* 139, 161.

Hetherington, M. J. & Ladd (2020). *Destroying trust in the media, science, and government has left America vulnerable to disaster.* The Brookings Institution. https://www.brookings.edu/blog/fixgov/2020/05/01/destroying-trust-in-the-media-science-and-government-has-left-america-vulnerable-to-disaster/

Hetherington, M. J., & Nelson, M. (2003). Anatomy of a rally effect: George W. Bush and the war on terrorism. *Political Science & Politics*, 36, 37–42.

Hodges, A. (2017). Trump's Formulaic Twitter Insults. *Anthropology News*, 58(1), e206-e210.

Holder, J. (2021). *Tracking Coronavirus Vaccinations Around the World*. The New York Times. https://www.nytimes.com/interactive/2021/world/covid-vaccinations-tracker.html

Hootsuite & We Are Social. (2020, October 27). *Digital 2020 October Statshot Report*. Hootsuite. https://blog.hootsuite.com/social-media-users-pass-4-billion/

Houseman, M. (2012). Pushing Ritual Frames Past Bateson. *Journal of Ritual Studies*, 26(2), 1-5.

Hsieh, H. F., & Shannon, S. E. (2005). Three approaches to qualitative content analysis. *Qualitative health research*, 15(9), 1277-1288.

Hswen, Y., Xu, X., Hing, A., Hawkins, J. B., Brownstein, J. S., & Gee, G. C. (2021). Association of "# covid19" Versus "# chinesevirus" With Anti-Asian Sentiments on Twitter: March 9–23, 2020. *American Journal of Public Health*, (0), e1-e9.

Information Resources Inc [IRI] (2020, April 23). *COVID-19 Impact: Consumer Spending Tracker for Measured Channels*. IRI. https://www.iriworldwide.com/IRI/media/Library/2020-04-30-IRI-BCG-COVID-Global-Consumer-Spend-Tracker.pdf

International Labour Office, International Organization for Migration & Office of the United Nations High Commissioner for Human Rights (2001). *International Migration, International Migration, Racism, Discrimination and Xenophobia*. The UN Refugee Agency. https://www.refworld.org/docid/49353b4d2.html,%20page%202

Islentyeva, A. (2020). On the Front Line in the Fight against the Virus: Conceptual Framing and War Patterns in Political Discourse. *Yearbook of the German Cognitive Linguistics Association*, 8(1), 157-180.

Iyengar, P. (2002). News framing as a multiparadigmatic research program: A response to Entman. *Journal of communication*, 52(4), 870-888.

Iyengar, S. (1990). The accessibility bias in politics: Television news and public opinion. *International Journal of Public Opinion Research*, 2(1), 1-15.

Jeung, R., Yellow Horse, A., Tara Popovic, T. & Lim R. (2021, March 16). *STOP AAPI HATE NATIONAL REPORT*. Stop AAPI Hate. https://secureservercdn.net/104.238.69.231/a1w.90d.myftpupload.com/wp-content/uploads/2021/03/210312-Stop-AAPI-Hate-National-Report-.pdf

Johnson, B. (2020, March 23). *Prime Minister's statement on coronavirus (COVID-19): 23 March 2020*. Gov. UK. https://www.gov.uk/government/speeches/pm-address-to-the-nation-on-coronavirus-23-march-2020

Jorge, A. (2020). *Hydroxychloroquine in the prevention of COVID-19 mortality*. The Lancet Rheumatology. https://www.thelancet.com/journals/lanrhe/article/PIIS2665-9913(20)30390-8/fulltext

Judd, E. (2020, March 2). *Crooked, Crazy, Crying: Trump's top nicknames for opponents*. Alarabiya News. https://english.alarabiya.net/features/2020/03/02/Crooked-Crazy-Crying-Trump-s-top-nicknames-for-opponents

Junk, J. & Peez, A. (2020, November 3). *The Populist Pandemic Playbook: COVID-19 and the Limits of Right-Wing Populist Government*. PRIF Blog. https://blog.prif.org/2020/11/03/the-populist-pandemic-playbook-covid-19-and-the-limits-of-right-wing-populist-government/

Jürgens, P., & Stark, B. (2017). The Power of Default on Reddit: A General Model to Measure the Influence of Information Intermediaries. *Policy & Internet*, 9(4), 395–419.

Kayam, O. (2018). Donald Trump's rhetoric: How an anti-political strategy helped him win the presidency. *Language and Dialogue*, 8(2), 183-208.

Keane, M., & Neal, T. (2021). Consumer panic in the COVID-19 pandemic. *Journal of econometrics*, 220(1), 86-105.

Kellner, D. (2016). *American nightmare: Donald Trump, media spectacle, and authoritarian populism* (Vol. 117). Springer.

Kemp, S. (2020, October 27). *Digital 2020 October Statshot Report*. https://datareportal.com/reports/digital-2020-october-global-statshot

Kinder, D. R., & Sanders, L. M. (1990). Mimicking political debate with survey questions: The case of white opinion on affirmative action for blacks. *Social cognition*, 8(1), 73-103.

Kinder, D. R., & Sanders, L. M. (1996). Framing the Issue: Elite Discourse and Popular Understanding; The Electoral Temptations of Race; Benign Neglect and Racial Codewords in the 1988 Presidential Campaign.

Kounang, N. (2020, February 7). *President Trump tweeted the coronavirus could weaken as weather warms. Scientists say it's too early to know*. CNN. https://edition.cnn.com/2020/02/07/health/trump-coronavirus-weaker-warm-weather/index.html

Kreis, R. (2017). The "tweet politics" of President Trump. *Journal of language and politics*, 16(4), 607-618.

Krippendorff, K. (2017). Three concepts to retire. *Annals of the international communication association,* 41(1), 92-99.

Krishnakumar, P. (2021, March 18). *Why hate crime data can't capture the true scope of anti-Asian violence*. CNN https://edition.cnn.com/2021/03/18/us/hate-crime-reporting-anti-asian-violence/index.html

Kyle, J., & Meyer, B. (2020). High Tide? Populism in Power, 1990-2020. Working Paper. Tony Blair Institute.

Ladkin, D. (2020). What Donald Trump's response to COVID-19 teaches us: it's time for our romance with leaders to end. *Leadership*, 16(3), 273-278.

LaFree, G., & Adamczyk, A. (2017). The impact of the Boston marathon bombings on public willingness to cooperate with police. *Justice quarterly*, 34(3), 459-490.

Lakoff (2016, July 23). *Understanding Trump*. George Lakoff. https://georgelakoff.com/2016/07/23/understanding-trump-2/

Lakoff, G. (2012). Explaining embodied cognition results. *Topics in cognitive science*, 4(4), 773-785.

Lakoff, G. (2014). *The all new don't think of an elephant!: Know your values and frame the debate.* Chelsea Green Publishing.

Lakoff, G. (2017, April 18). *Read our full conversation with George Lakoff on "your brain on Trump"*. Marketplace. https://www.marketplace.org/2017/04/18/transcript-blog-trump-george-lakoff/

Lakoff, G. (2018, May 24). *How You Help Trump*. FrameLab. https://medium.com/@GeorgeLakoff/how-you-help-trump-9d0139b9d4c9

Lenthang, M. (2021, March 11). *Asian American mother spit on, called 'Chinese virus' while holding baby*. Abc News. https://abcnews.go.com/US/asian-american-mother-spit-called-chinese-virus-holding/story?id=76387423

Lerner, B. H. (2003). *The breast cancer wars: hope, fear, and the pursuit of a cure in twentieth-century America*. New York: Oxford University Press.

Lewandowsky, S., Jetter, M., & Ecker, U. K. (2020). Using the president's tweets to understand political diversion in the age of social media. *Nature communications*, 11(1), 1-12.

Link, B. G., & Phelan, J. C. (2001). Conceptualizing stigma. *Annual review of Sociology*, 27(1), 363-385.

Linstrom, M., & Marais, W. (2012). Qualitative news frame analysis: A methodology. *Communitas*, 17, 21-38.

Lovelace, J. B., & Hunter, S. T. (2013). Charismatic, ideological, and pragmatic leaders' influence on subordinate creative performance across the creative process. *Creativity Research Journal*, 25(1), 59-74.

Lule, J. (2019). News Language and Framing: Return of the Repressed in Media Studies. In: D'Angelo, P., Lule, J., Neuman, W. R., Rodriguez, L., Dimitrova, D. V., & Carragee, K. M. (2019). Beyond framing: A forum for framing researchers. *Journalism & mass communication quarterly*, 96(1), 12-30.

Macilwain, C. (2015). Change the cancer conversation. *Nature*, 520(7545), 7-7.

Macron E. (2020, March 16). *ADRESSE AUX FRANÇAIS DU PRÉSIDENT DE LA RÉPUBLIQUE EMMANUEL MACRON*. Elysee. https://www.elysee.fr/emmanuel-macron/2020/03/16/adresse-aux-francais-covid19

Malouf, J. (2020, May 8). *Scorekeeping With Donald Trump in a COVID-19 Language Game*. E-international Relations. https://www.e-ir.info/2020/05/08/scorekeeping-with-donald-trump-in-a-covid-19-language-game/

Manfredi-Sánchez, J. L., Amado-Suárez, A., & Waisbord, S. (2021). Presidential Twitter in the Face of COVID-19: Between Populism and Pop Politics. *Comunicar: Media Education Research Journal*, 29(66), 79-90.

Mannion, R., & Speed, E. (2021). Populism, pestilence and plague in the time of coronavirus. *International Journal of Human Rights in Healthcare*.

Matthes, J. (2008). Media frames and public opinion: Exploring the boundaries of framing effects in a two-wave panel study. *Studies in Communication Sciences*, 8(2), 101-128.

Matthes, J., & Kohring, M. (2008). The content analysis of media frames: Toward improving reliability and validity. *Journal of communication*, 58(2), 258-279.

Mayring, P. (2000). Qualitative content analysis. *Forum: Qualitative Social Research*, 1(2).

McCarthy, M., & Carter, R. (2004). "There's millions of them": hyperbole in everyday conversation. *Journal of pragmatics*, 36(2), 149-184.

McCauley, M., Minsky, S., & Viswanath, K. (2013). The H1N1 pandemic: media frames, stigmatization and coping. *BMC Public Health*, 13(1), 1116.

McCloskey, J. (2021, February 26). *Racists screamed 'Ching Chong... Chinese virus' at Asian man while beating him up.* Metro. https://metro.co.uk/2021/02/25/racists-screamed-ching-chong-chinese-virus-at-asian-man-beating-him-14145928/

McGraw, T. (2020, December 7). *Spending* 2020 *Together on Twitter*. Twitter. https://blog.twitter.com/en_us/topics/insights/2020/spending-2020-together-on-twitter.html

McPherson, M., Smith-Lovin, L., & Cook, J. M. (2001). Birds of a feather: Homophily in social networks. *Annual review of sociology*, 27(1), 415-444.

Medaris Miller, A. (2020, October 6). *Coronavirus survivors and families of victims react to Trump's message: 'You do not have a choice if COVID-19 dominates your life'*. The Insider. https://www.businessinsider.com/covid-survivors-bereaved-react-to-trumps-message-insulting-disrespectful-dangerous-2020-10?r=DE&IR=T

Meeks, L. (2020). Defining the Enemy: How Donald Trump Frames the News Media. *Journalism & Mass Communication Quarterly*, 97(1), 211-234.

Mendoza-Denton, N. (2020). 5 Part II Introduction: The Show Must Go On: Hyperbole and Falsehood in Trump's Performance. *Language in the Trump Era: Scandals and Emergencies*, 91.

Meyer, B. (2020). *Pandemic Populism: An Analysis of Populist Leaders' Responses to Covid-19*. London: Tony Blair Institute for Global Change.

Milla, M. N., Putra, I. E., & Umam, A. N. (2019). Stories from jihadists: Significance, identity, and radicalization through the call for jihad. *Peace and Conflict*, 25, 111–121.

Mills, S. (2003). Caught between sexism, anti-sexism andpolitical correctness': feminist women's negotiations with naming practices. *Discourse & Society*, 14(1), 87-11

Mint (2020, January 9). *Won't be silenced: Trump after Twitter's permanent ban.* Mint. https://www.livemint.com/news/world/wont-be-silenced-trump-after-twitter-s-permanent-ban-11610161192704.html.

Mudde, C., & Kaltwasser, C. R. (2017). *Populism: A very short introduction*. Oxford University Press.

Mueller, J. E. (1970). Presidential popularity from Truman to Johnson. *The American Political Science Review*, 64, 18–33.

Müller, J. W. (2017). *What is populism?*. University of Pennsylvania Press.

Mutua, S. N., & Oloo Ong'ong'a, D. (2020). Online news media framing of COVID-19 pandemic: Probing the initial phases of the disease outbreak in international media. *European Journal of Interactive Multimedia and Education*, 1(2), e02006.

Mutua, S. N., & Ong'ong'a, D. O. (2020). Online News Media Framing of COVID-19 Pandemic: Probing the Initial Phases of the Disease Outbreak in International Media.

NBCNews. (2020). *Twitter removes tweet highlighted by Trump falsely claiming COVID-19 'cure'.* NBC News. https://www.nbcnews.com/politics/donald-trump/twitter-removes-tweet-highlighted-trump-falsely-claiming-covid-cure-n1235075

Neuman, W. R. (2019). The Future of Framing Research. In: D'Angelo, P., Lule, J., Neuman, W. R., Rodriguez, L., Dimitrova, D. V., & Carragee, K. M. (2019). Beyond framing: A forum for framing researchers. *Journalism & mass communication quarterly*, 96(1), 12-30.

Neuman, W. R., Neuman, R. W., Just, M. R., & Crigler, A. N. (1992). *Common knowledge: News and the construction of political meaning.* University of Chicago Press.

new left. Berkeley, CA: University of California Press.

Nielsen, R. K., Fletcher, R., Newman, N., Brennen, S. J., & Howard, P. N. (2020). *Navigating the 'infodemic': How people in six countries access and rate news and information about coronavirus*. Reuters Institute. https://reutersinstitute.politics.ox.ac.uk/infodemic-how-people-six-countries-access-and-rate-news-and-information-about-coronavirus

Nielson, S. & Woodword, A. (2020, December 24). *A comprehensive timeline of the coronavirus pandemic at 1 year, from China's first case to the present*. Business Insider. https://www.businessinsider.com/coronavirus-pandemic-timeline-history-major-events-2020-3?r=DE&IR=T

Nordin, M. Z. F. (2018). The identity in religious language in Malaysia. *American Journal of Humanities and Social Sciences Research*, 12(8), 74-78.

Nwakpu, E. S., Ezema, V. O., & Ogbodo, J. N. (2020). Nigeria media framing of coronavirus pandemic and audience response. *Health Promotion Perspectives*, 10(3), 192.

Nyhan, B., & Reifler, J. (2010). When corrections fail: The persistence of political misperceptions. *Political Behavior*, 32(2), 303-330.

Ogbodo, J. N., Onwe, E. C., Chukwu, J., Nwasum, C. J., Nwakpu, E. S., Nwankwo, S. U., ... & Ogbaeja, N. I. (2020). Communicating health crisis: a content analysis of global media framing of COVID-19. *Health Promotion Perspectives*, 10(3), 257.

Okano-Heijmans, M. (2020). *Coronavirus: The World's First Digital Pandemic*. Clingendael Institute of International Relations. https://www. clingendael. org/publication/coronavirus-worlds-first-digital-pandemic

Oliver, J. E., & Rahn, W. M. (2016). Rise of the Trumpenvolk: Populism in the 2016 Election. *The ANNALS of the American Academy of Political and Social Science*, 667(1), 189-206.

Oltermann P. (2020, April 16). *Angela Merkel draws on science background in Covid-19 explainer*. The Guardian. https://www.theguardian.com/world/2020/apr/16/angela-merkel-draws-on-science-background-in-covid-19-explainer-lockdown-exit

Ollstein, A. M. (2020, April 2). *Coronavirus quarantine, travel ban could backfire, experts fear.* Politico. https://www.politico.com/news/2020/02/04/coronavirus-quaratine-travel-110750

Pan, Z. & Kosicki, G.M. (1993). Framing analysis: an approach to news discourse. *Political Communication* 10: 55-76.

Pan, Z., & Kosicki, G. M. (1993). Framing analysis: An approach to news discourse. Political communication, 10(1), 55-75.Pan, Z., & Kosicki, G. M. (1993). Framing analysis: An approach to news discourse. *Political communication*, 10(1), 55-75.

Pariser, E. (2011). The filter bubble: What the Internet is hiding from you. New York, NY: Penguin Press.

Paulus, D. (2020, May 22). *Why German Leaders Refrained From Declaring 'War' on the Coronavirus*. The Conversation. https://theconversation.com/how-politicians-talk-about-coronavirus-in-germany-where-war-metaphors-are-avoided-137427

Pei, S., Kandula, S., & Shaman, J. (2020). Differential effects of intervention timing on COVID-19 spread in the United States. *Science advances*, 6(49), eabd6370.

Pew Research Center (2020). About seven-in-ten US adults say they need to take breaks from COVID-19 news. Washington, DC: Pew Research Center, 1-5.

Platow, M. J., Van Knippenberg, D., Haslam, S. A., Van Knippenberg, B., & Spears, R. (2006). A special gift we bestow on you for being representative of us: Considering leader charisma from a self-categorization perspective. *British Journal of Social Psychology*, 45(2), 303-320.

Pluwak, A. (2013). An Analysis of the War Against the Disease-Metaphor in Selected 2011 Presidential Speeches of Felipe Calderon. *Cognitive Studies| Études cognitives*, (13), 237-260.

Powers, M. (2014). The structural organization of NGO publicity work: Explaining divergent publicity strategies at humanitarian and human rights organizations. *International journal of communication*, 8, 18.

Price, V., Tewksbury, D., & Powers, E. (1997). Switching trains of thought: The impact of news frames on readers' cognitive responses. *Communication research*, 24(5), 481-506.

Rajandran, K. (2020). 'A Long Battle Ahead': Malaysian and Singaporean Prime Ministers Employ War Metaphors for COVID-19. *GEMA Online® Journal of Language Studies*, 20(3).

Rand, D.(2020, November 2). *Revealed: Joe Biden has been hit harder by Twitter's new retweet policy than Donald Trump*. NewStatesman https://www.newstatesman.com/world/2020/11/revealed-joe-biden-has-been-hit-harder-twitter-s-new-retweet-policy-donald-trump

Redfield. R. (2020, December 3). *A Conversation with CDC Director Dr. Robert. U.S. Chamber of Commerce Foundation* [Video]. Youtube. https://www.youtube.com/watch?v=3BAVCKNeHAc&%3Bfeature=emb_title&ab_channel=U.S.ChamberofCommerceFoundation

Redlener, I., Sachs, J. D., Hansen, S., & Hupert, N. (2020). *130,000-210,000 Avoidable Covid-19 Deaths—And Counting—In the US*. New York: National Center for Disaster Preparedness, Columbia University. https://ncdp.columbia.edu/custom-content/uploads/2020/10/Avoidable-COVID-19-Deaths-US-NCDP.pdf

Reese, S. D. (2007). The framing project: A bridging model for media research revisited. *Journal of communication*, 57(1), 148-154.

Reese, S. D. (2010). *Finding frames in a web of culture: The case of the war on terror. In Doing news framing analysis* (pp. 33-58). Routledge.

Reese, S. D., Gandy Jr, O. H., & Grant, A. E. (Eds.). (2001). *Framing public life: Perspectives on media and our understanding of the social world*. Routledge.

Relman, D. A. (2020, April 7). *Rapid Expert Consultation on SARS-CoV-2 Survival in Relation to Temperature and Humidity and Potential for Seasonality for the COVID-19 Pandemic*. National Academies of Sciences, Engineering, and Medicine. https://www.nap.edu/catalog/25771/rapid-expert-consultation-on-sars-cov-2-survival-in-relation-to-temperature-and-humidity-and-potential-for-seasonality-for-the-covid-19-pandemic-april-7-202

0

Reuters (2020a). *Timeline: How the global coronavirus pandemic unfolded*. Reuters. https://www.reuters.com/article/us-health-coronavirus-timeline-idUSKBN26K0AQ

Ribeiro, B., Hartley, S., Nerlich, B., & Jaspal, R. (2018). Media coverage of the Zika crisis in Brazil: the construction of a 'war' frame that masked social and gender inequalities. *Social Science & Medicine*, 200, 137-144.

Rice-Oxley, M. & Kalia, A. (2018). *How to spot a populist*. The Guardian. https://www.theguardian.com/news/2018/dec/03/what-is-populism-trump-farage-orban-bolsonaro

Rosenberg, C. E., & Golden, J. L. (Eds.). (1992). *Framing disease: studies in cultural history*. Rutgers University Press.

Rosenberg, H., Syed, S., & Rezaie, S. (2020). The Twitter pandemic: The critical role of Twitter in the dissemination of medical information and misinformation during the COVID-19 pandemic. *Canadian Journal of Emergency Medicine*, 1-4.

Ross, A. S., & Caldwell, D. (2020). 'Going negative': An appraisal analysis of the rhetoric of Donald Trump on Twitter. *Language & communication*, 70, 13-27.

Ross, A. S., & Rivers, D. J. (2020). Donald Trump, legitimisation and a new political rhetoric. *World Englishes*, 39(4), 623-637.

Rufai, S. R., & Bunce, C. (2020). World leaders' usage of Twitter in response to the COVID-19 pandemic: a content analysis. *Journal of Public Health*, 42(3), 510-516.

Ruiz, N., Mensace Horowitz, J. & Tamir, C. (2020, July 1). *Many Black and Asian Americans Say They Have Experienced Discrimination Amid the COVID-19 Outbreak.* The Pew Research Center. https://www.pewresearch.org/social-trends/2020/07/01/many-black-and-asian-americans-say-they-have-experienced-discrimination-amid-the-covid-19-outbreak/

Rupar, A. (2020, January 8*). How Trump's speech led to the Capitol.* Vox News. https://www.vox.com/22220746/trump-speech-incite-capitol-riot

Rutledge, P. E. (2020). Trump, COVID-19, and the War on Expertise. *The American Review of Public Administration*, 50(6-7), 505-511.

Schaffner, B. F., & Sellers, P. J. (Eds.). (2009). *Winning with words: the origins and impact of political framing*. Routledge.

Schaeffer, K. (2020, July 24). *A look at the Americans who believe there is some truth to the conspiracy theory that COVID-19 was planned.* The Pew Research Center. https://www.pewresearch.org/fact-tank/2020/07/24/a-look-at-the-americans-who-believe-there-is-some-truth-to-the-conspiracy-theory-that-covid-19-was-planned/

Scheufele, D. A., & Iyengar, S. (2012*). The state of framing research: A call for new directions. The Oxford Handbook of Political Communication Theories*. New York: Oxford University Press, 1-26.

Schroeder, R. (2018). *Social Theory after the Internet: Media, Technology, and Globalization*. London: UCL Press.

Science News (2020, December 11). *This COVID-19 pandemic timeline shows how fast the coronavirus took over our lives*. Science News. https://www.sciencenews.org/article/coronavirus-covid19-pandemic-timeline-events

Select Subcommittee on the Coronavirus Crisis (2020, October 2). *Select Subcommittee Analysis Shows Pattern Of Political Interference By The Trump Administration In Coronavirus Response.* House of Representatives. https://coronavirus.house.gov/news/press-releases/select-subcommittee-analysis-shows-pattern-political-interference-trump

Semetko, H. A., & Valkenburg, P. M. (2000). Framing European politics: A content analysis of press and television news. *Journal of communication*, 50(2), 93-109.

Senge, P. M. (1990). *The art and practice of the learning organization*. New York: Currency Doubleday.

Shafer, J. G. (2017). Donald Trump's "political incorrectness": Neoliberalism as frontstage racism on social media. *Social Media+ Society*, 3(3), 1-10.

Shah, D. V., McLeod, D. M., Rojas, H., Cho, J., Wagner, M. W., & Friedland, L. A. (2017). Revising the communication mediation model for a new political communication ecology. *Human Communication Research*, 43(4), 491-504.

Shoichet E. C. (2020, February 7). *The US coronavirus travel ban could backfire. Here's how.* CNN. https://edition.cnn.com/2020/02/07/health/coronavirus-travel-ban/index.html

Shaw, M. E. M. D. L., Weaver, D. H., & Mc Combs, M. (1997*). Communication and democracy: Exploring the intellectual frontiers in agenda-setting theory*. Psychology Press.

Shear, D. M. & Mervosh, S. (2020, April 23). *Trump Encourages Protest Against Governors Who Have Imposed Virus Restrictions.* The New York Times. https://www.nytimes.com/2020/04/17/us/politics/trump-coronavirus-governors.html

Shear, D. M., Haberman, M., Weiland, N., LaFraniere, S. & Mazzetti, M. (2020, December 31. Trump's Focus as the Pandemic Raged: What Would It Mean for Him?. The New York Times. https://www.nytimes.com/2020/12/31/us/politics/trump-coronavirus.html

Shurafa, C., Darwish, K., & Zaghouani, W. (2020, October). Political Framing: US COVID19 Blame Game. In International Conference on Social Informatics (pp. 333-351). Springer, Cham.

Simon, A., & Xenos, M. (2000). Media framing and effective public deliberation. *Political communication*, 17(4), 363-376.

Slothuus, R. (2008). More than weighting cognitive importance: A dual-process model of issue framing effects. *Political Psychology*, 29(1), 1-28.

Slothuus, R., & De Vreese, C. H. (2010). Political parties, motivated reasoning, and issue framing effects. *The Journal of Politics*, 72(3), 630-645.

Smith, C. (2020, April 9). *Scientists warn that Trump is wrong: Warm weather won't kill coronavirus.* BGR. https://bgr.com/science/coronavirus-usa-warmer-weather-wont-reduce-covid-19-transmission-5815724/

Sniderman, P. M., & Theriault, S. M. (2004). The structure of political argument and the logic of issue framing. *Studies in public opinion: Attitudes, nonattitudes, measurement error, and change*, 133-65.

Snow, D. A., Rochford Jr, E. B., Worden, S. K., & Benford, R. D. (1986). Frame alignment processes, micromobilization, and movement participation. *American sociological review*, 464-481.

Snow, D. A., Vliegenthart, R., & Corrigall-Brown, C. (2007). Framing the French riots: A comparative study of frame variation. *Social forces*, 86(2), 385-415.

Solender, A. (2020, May 22). *All The Times Trump Has Promoted Hydroxychloroquine*. The Guardian. https://www.forbes.com/sites/andrewsolender/2020/05/22/all-the-times-trump-promoted-hydroxychloroquine/

Solomon, W. S. (1992). News frames and media packages: Covering El Salvador. *Critical Studies in Media Communication*, 9(1), 56-74.

Somerville, J. (1981). Patriotism and war. *Ethics*, 91, 568–578.

Sondermann, E., & Ulbert, C. (2020). The threat of thinking in threats: reframing global health during and after COVID-19. *Zeitschrift für Friedens-und Konfliktforschung*, 9(2), 309-320.

Sontag, S. (1978). *Illness as metaphor*. Farrar, Straus and Giroux.

Stark, B., Stegmann, D., Magin, M., & Jürgens, P. (2020). *Are algorithms a threat to democracy? The rise of intermediaries: A challenge for public discourse*. AlgorithmWatch. https://algorithmwatch.org/en/wp-content/uploads/2020/05/Governing-Platforms-communications-study-Stark-May-2020-AlgorithmWatch.pdf

Steffens, N. K., & Haslam, S. A. (2013). Power through 'us': Leaders' use of we-referencing language predicts election victory. *PloS one*, 8(10), e77952.

Steier, F. (2013). Gregory Bateson gets a mobile phone. *Mobile Media & Communication*, 1(1), 160-165.

Sturla, A., Alsharif, M., Sgueglia, K., Ly, L. & CNN (2021, February 28). *Attacks against people of Asian descent are on the rise in NYC. The city is pushing to combat it*. CNN. https://edition.cnn.com/2021/02/27/us/new-york-initiative-anti-asian-attacks/index.html

Swindells, K. (2020, November 2). *Revealed: Joe Biden has been hit harder by Twitter's new retweet policy than Donald Trump*. NewStatesman https://www.newstatesman.com/world/2020/11/revealed-joe-biden-has-been-hit-harder-twitter-s-new-retweet-policy-donald-trump

Taggart, P. A., & Parkin, F. (2000). *Populism*. Open University Press.

Taras, D. (2019). *Political Leaders and Social Media: An Introduction. In Power Shift? Political Leadership and Social Media* (pp. 1-14). Routledge.

Taylor, B. D. (2021, March 17). *A Timeline of the Coronavirus Pandemic.* The New York Times. https://www.nytimes.com/article/coronavirus-timeline.html

Tedros, A. G., (2020, March 11). *WHO Director-General's opening remarks at the media briefing on COVID-19. World Health Organization.* https://www.who.int/director-general/speeches/detail/who-director-general-s-opening-remarks-at-the-media-briefing-on-covid-19---11-march-2020

Tesch, R. (2013). *Qualitative research: Analysis types and software*. Routledge.

The Wall Steert Journal (2020). *Trump Claim That Malaria Drugs Treat Coronavirus Sparks Warnings, Shortages*. https://www.wsj.com/articles/trump-claim-that-malaria-drugs-treat-coronavirus-sparks-warnings-shortages-11584981897

Theye, K., & Melling, S. (2018). Total losers and bad hombres: The political incorrectness and perceived authenticity of Donald J. Trump. *Southern Communication Journal*, 83(5), 322-337.

Thomas, T., Wilson, A., Tonkin, E., Miller, E. R., & Ward, P. R. (2020). How the media places responsibility for the COVID-19 pandemic–An Australian media analysis. *Frontiers in public health*, 8, 483.

Thomas, Z. (2020, February 13). *WHO says fake coronavirus claims causing 'infodemic'.* BBC. https://www.bbc.com/news/technology-51497800

Thorbecke, C. (2021, February 25). *California commits $1.4 million to combat 'horrific' attacks on Asian Americans*. Abc News. https://abcnews.go.com/US/california-commits-14-million-combat-horrific-attacks-asian/story?id=76084993

Tolefson, G. (2020, October 5). *How Trump damaged science — and why it could take decades to recover*. nature. https://www.nature.com/articles/d41586-020-02800-9

Turse, N. (2020, March 5). *As Trump stumbles on coronavirus, health experts warn against border closure.* The Intercept. https://theintercept.com/2020/03/05/coronavirus-trump-closing-borders/

Trump, D. (2019, June 17). *Transcript: ABC News' George Stephanopoulos' exclusive interview with President Trump.* ABC News. https://abcnews.go.com/Politics/transcript-abc-news-george-stephanopoulos-exclusive-interview-president/story?id=63749144

Trump, D. (2020, October 26). *The 60 Minutes interview that President Trump cut short.* CBS News. https://www.cbsnews.com/news/president-trump-60-minutes-interview-lesley-stahl/

Trump, D. [Reuters]. (2020, October 8). *Trump calls his illness 'a blessing from god,' vows experimental drugs for all* [Video]. Youtube. https://www.youtube.com/watch?v=Ee2WWEqP4L4&t=45s

Trump, D. [Global News] (2020, October 19). *Coronavirus: Trump says U.S. would see massive depression if he "listened totally to the scientists"* [Video]. Youtube. https://www.youtube.com/watch?v=mHEpFvBrEV8

Trump, D. [The Telegraph] (2020, March 23a). *President Trump says he is a 'wartime president' battling an 'invisible enemy' over coronavirus* [Video].Youtube. https://www.youtube.com/watch?v=vOe4Ksoa5bk

Trump, D. [@realDonaldTrump]. (2020, February 28b). *The Do Nothing Democrats were busy wasting time on the Immigration Hoax, & anything else they could do to make the Republican Party look bad, while I was busy calling early BORDER & FLIGHT closings, putting us way ahead in our battle with Coronavirus. Dems called it VERY wrong!* [Tweet]. Trump archiver. https://bit.ly/3syCKue

Trump, D. [@realDonaldTrump]. (2020, February 25b). *Democrats talking point is that we are doing badly. If the virus disappeared tomorrow, they would say we did a really poor, and even incompetent, job. Not fair, but it is what it is. So far, by the way, we have not had one death. Let's keep it that way!* [Tweet]. Trump archiver. https://bit.ly/3syCKue

Trump, D. [@realDonaldTrump]. (2020, February 25a). *Cryin' Chuck Schumer is complaining, for publicity purposes only, that I should be asking for more money than $2.5 Billion to prepare for Coronavirus. If I asked for more he would say it is too much. He didn't like my early travel closings. I was right. He is incompetent!* [Tweet]. Trump archiver. https://bit.ly/3syCKue

Trump, D. [@realDonaldTrump]. (2020, March 5a). *I NEVER said people that are feeling sick should go to work. This is just more Fake News and disinformation put out by the Democrats, in particular MSDNC. Comcast covers the CoronaVirus situation horribly, only looking to do harm to the incredible & successful effort being made!* [Tweet]. Trump archiver. https://bit.ly/3syCKue

Trump, D. [@realDonaldTrump]. (2020, March 5b). *With approximately 100,000 CoronaVirus cases worldwide, and 3,280 deaths, the United States, because of quick action on closing our borders, has, as of now, only 129 cases (40 Americans brought in) and 11 deaths. We are working very hard to keep these numbers as low as possible*! [Tweet]. Trump archiver. https://bit.ly/3syCKue

Trump, D. [@realDonaldTrump]. (2020, March 5c). *I NEVER said people that are feeling sick should go to work. This is just more Fake News and disinformation put out by the Democrats, in particular MSDNC. Comcast covers the CoronaVirus situation horribly, only looking to do harm to the incredible & successful effort being made!* [Tweet]. Trump archiver. https://bit.ly/3syCKue

Trump, D. [@realDonaldTrump]. (2020, January 24). *China has been working very hard to contain the Coronavirus. The United States greatly appreciates their efforts and transparency. It will all work out well. In particular, on behalf of the American People, I want to thank President Xi!* [Tweet]. Trump archiver. https://bit.ly/3syCKue

Trump, D. [@realDonaldTrump]. (2020, January 27). *We are in very close communication with China concerning the virus. Very few cases reported in USA, but strongly on watch. We have offered China and President Xi any help that is necessary. Our experts are extraordinary!* [Tweet]. Trump archiver. https://bit.ly/3syCKue

Trump, D. [@realDonaldTrump]. (2020, January 30). *Working closely with China and others on Coronavirus outbreak. Only 5 people in U.S., all in good recovery* [Tweet]. Trump archiver. https://bit.ly/3syCKue

Trump, D. [@realDonaldTrump]. (2020, January 29). *Just received a briefing on the Coronavirus in China from all of our GREAT agencies, who are also working closely with China. We will continue to monitor the ongoing developments. We have the best experts anywhere in the world, and they are on top of it 24/7! https://t.co/rrtF1Stk78* [Tweet]. Trump archiver. https://bit.ly/3syCKue

Trump, D. [@realDonaldTrump]. (2020, February 7a). *Just had a long and very good conversation by phone with President Xi of China. He is strong, sharp and powerfully focused on leading the counterattack on the Coronavirus. He feels they are doing very well, even building hospitals in a matter of only days. Nothing is easy, but* [Tweet]. Trump archiver. https://bit.ly/3syCKue

Trump, D. [@realDonaldTrump]. (2020, February 7b). *he will be successful, especially as the weather starts to warm & the virus hopefully becomes weaker, and then gone. Great discipline is taking place in China, as President Xi strongly leads what will be a very successful operation. We are working closely with China to help!* [Tweet]. Trump archiver. https://bit.ly/3syCKue

Trump, D. [@realDonaldTrump]. (2020, February 27a). *Congratulations and thank you to our great Vice President & all of the many professionals doing such a fine job at CDC & all other agencies on the Coronavirus situation. Only a very small number in U.S., & China numbers look to be going down. All countries working well together!* [Tweet]. Trump archiver. https://bit.ly/3syCKue

Trump, D. [@realDonaldTrump]. (2020, February 27b). "*Diagnosis positive: @CNN is infected with Trump Derangement Syndrome. I'm calling out CNN for irresponsibly politicizing what should be a unifying battle against a virus that doesn't choose sides." @trish_regan @FoxNews Like I say, they are Fake News!* [Tweet]. Trump archiver. https://bit.ly/3syCKue

Trump, D. [@realDonaldTrump]. (2020, February 24). *The Coronavirus is very much under control in the USA. We are in contact with everyone and all relevant countries. CDC & World Health have been working hard and very smart. Stock Market starting to look very good to me!* [Tweet]. Trump archiver. https://bit.ly/3syCKue

Trump, D. [@realDonaldTrump]. (2020, February 28a). *So, the Coronavirus, which started in China and spread to various countries throughout the world, but very slowly in the U.S. because President Trump closed our border, and ended flights, VERY EARLY, is now being blamed, by the Do Nothing Democrats, to be the fault of "Trump"* [Tweet]. Trump archiver. https://bit.ly/3syCKue

Trump, D. [@realDonaldTrump]. (2020, July 15). *...campaign. Both were heavily involved in our historic 2016 win, and I look forward to having a big and very important second win together. This one should be a lot easier as our poll numbers are rising fast, the economy is getting better, vaccines and therapeutics will soon...*[Tweet]. Trump archiver. https://bit.ly/3syCKue

Trump, D. [@realDonaldTrump]. (2020, July 21a). *You will never hear this on the Fake News concerning the China Virus, but by comparison to most other countries, who are suffering greatly, we are doing very well - and we have done things that few other countries could have done!* [Tweet]. Trump archiver. https://bit.ly/3syCKue

Trump, D. [@realDonaldTrump]. (2020, July 21b). *Tremendous progress being made on Vaccines and Therapeutics!!!* [Tweet]. Trump archiver. https://bit.ly/3syCKue

Trump, D. [@realDonaldTrump]. (2020, July 27). *....would destroy our American cities, and worse, if Sleepy Joe Biden, the puppet of the Left, ever won. Markets would crash* *and cities would burn. Our Country would suffer like never before. We will beat the Virus, soon, and go on to the Golden Age - better than ever before!* [Tweet]. Trump archiver. https://bit.ly/3syCKue

Trump, D. [@realDonaldTrump]. (2020, July 27). *....would destroy our American cities, and worse, if Sleepy Joe Biden, the puppet of the Left, ever won. Markets would crash and cities would burn. Our Country would suffer like never before. We will beat the Virus, soon, and go on to the Golden Age - better than ever before!* [Tweet]. Trump archiver. https://bit.ly/3syCKue

Trump, D. [@realDonaldTrump]. (2020, August 3a) *In an illegal late night coup, Nevada's clubhouse Governor made it impossible for Republicans to win the state. Post Office could never handle the Traffic of Mail-In Votes without preparation. Using Covid to steal the state. See you in Court! https://t.co/cNSPINgCY7* [Tweet]. Trump archiver. https://bit.ly/3syCKue

Trump, D. [@realDonaldTrump]. (2020, August 3b). *With the exception of New York & a few other locations, we've done MUCH better than most other Countries in dealing with the China Virus. Many of these countries are now having a major second wave. The Fake News is working overtime to make the USA (& me) look as bad as possible!* [Tweet]. Trump archiver. https://bit.ly/3syCKue

Trump, D. [@realDonaldTrump]. (2020, August 7). *Pelosi and Schumer only interested in Bailout Money for poorly run Democrat cities and states. Nothing to do with China Virus! Want one trillion dollars. No interest. We are going a different way!* [Tweet]. Trump archiver. https://bit.ly/3syCKue

Trump, D. [@realDonaldTrump]. (2020, August 11). *More Testing, which is a good thing (we have the most in the world), equals more Cases, which is Fake News Gold. They use Cases to demean the incredible job being done by the great men & women of the U.S. fighting the China Plague!* [Tweet]. Trump archiver. https://bit.ly/3syCKue

Trump, D. [@realDonaldTrump]. (2020, August 22). *The deep state, or whoever, over at the FDA is making it very difficult for drug companies to get people in order to test the vaccines and therapeutics. Obviously, they are hoping to delay the answer until after November 3rd. Must focus on speed, and saving lives!* @SteveFDA [Tweet]. Trump archiver. https://bit.ly/3syCKue

Trump, D. [@realDonaldTrump]. (2020, September 3). *Sleepy Joe Hiden' was acknowledged by his own people to have done a terrible job on a much easier situation, H1N1 Swine Flu. The OBiden Administration failed badly on this, & now he sits back in his basement and criticizes every move we make on the China Virus. DOING GREAT JOB! https://t.co/p2H40mD7Sh* [Tweet]. Trump archiver. https://bit.ly/3syCKue

Trump, D. [@realDonaldTrump]. (2020, September 7). *Starting to get VERY high marks in our handling of the Coronavirus (China Virus), especially when compared to other countries and areas of the world. Now the Vaccines (Plus) are coming, and fast!* [Tweet]. Trump archiver. https://bit.ly/3syCKue

Trump, D. [@realDonaldTrump]. (2020, September 8). *Because of the China Virus, my Campaign, which has raised a lot of money, was forced to spend in order to counter the Fake News reporting about the way we handled it (China Ban, etc.). We did, and are doing, a GREAT job, and have a lot of money left over, much more than 2016....*[Tweet]. Trump archiver. https://bit.ly/3syCKue

Trump, D. [@realDonaldTrump]. (2020, September 10). *On November 3rd, Michigan will decide whether we will quickly return to record prosperity—or whether we allow Sleepy Joe Biden to impose a $4 TRILLION DOLLAR TAX HIKE, ban American Energy, confiscate your guns, shutdown the economy, shutdown auto production, delay* [Tweet]. Trump archiver. https://bit.ly/3syCKue

Trump, D. [@realDonaldTrump]. (2020, September 16). *Democrats are "heartless". They don't want to give STIMULUS PAYMENTS to people who desperately need the money, and whose fault it was NOT that the plague came in from China. Go for the much higher numbers, Republicans, it all comes back to the USA anyway (one way or another!)* [Tweet]. Trump archiver. https://bit.ly/3syCKue

Trump, D. [@realDonaldTrump]. (2020, September 23). *Big news. Numerous great companies are seeing fantastic results. @FDA must move quickly! https://t.co/2pDrmRPOxc* [Tweet]. Trump archiver. https://bit.ly/3syCKue

Trump, D. [@realDonaldTrump]. (2020, September 25). *Governor Andrew Cuomo of New York wants to put New York at the END of the Vaccine List in that he doesn't trust the @FDA or Federal Government, even though the Vaccines are being developed by the finest Labs in the World. Wish he trusted us on Nursing Homes!* [Tweet]. Trump archiver. https://bit.ly/3syCKue

Trump, D. [@realDonaldTrump]. (2020, September 30). *Many more people would have died from the China Virus if Sleepy Joe were your President. He didn't even want me to close our Country to Infected China until TWO MONTHS later, when he said I was right. Now he likes to say I didn't close up "fast enough". Just another politician!* [Tweet]. Trump archiver. https://bit.ly/3syCKue

Trump, D. [@realDonaldTrump]. (2020, October 3). *Doctors, Nurses and ALL at the GREAT Walter Reed Medical Center, and others from likewise incredible institutions who have joined them, are AMAZING!!!Tremendous progress has been made over the last 6 months in fighting this PLAGUE. With their help, I am feeling well!* [Tweet]. Trump archiver. https://bit.ly/3syCKue

Trump, D. [@realDonaldTrump]. (2020, October 5a). *....invincible hero, who not only survived every dirty trick the Democrats threw at him, but the Chinese virus as well. He will show America we no longer have to be afraid." @MirandaDevine @NYPost Thank you Miranda. Was over until the Plague came in from China. Will win anyway!* [Tweet]. Trump archiver. https://bit.ly/3syCKue

Trump, D. [@realDonaldTrump]. (2020, October 5b). *I will be leaving the great Walter Reed Medical Center today at 6:30 P.M. Feeling really good! Don't be afraid of Covid.*

*Don't let it dominate your life. We have developed, under the Trump Administration, some really great drugs & knowledge. I feel better than I did 20 years ago!* [Tweet]. Trump archiver. https://bit.ly/3syCKue

Trump, D. [@realDonaldTrump]. (2020, October 6a). *Flu season is coming up! Many people every year, sometimes over 100,000, and despite the Vaccine, die from the Flu. Are we going to close down our Country? No, we have learned to live with it, just like we are learning to live with Covid, in most populations far less lethal!!!* [Tweet]. Trump archiver. https://bit.ly/3syCKue

Trump, D. [@realDonaldTrump]. (2020, October 6b*)....also coming back in record numbers. We are leading the World in Economic Recovery, and THE BEST IS YET TO COME!* [Tweet]. Trump archiver. https://bit.ly/3syCKue

Trump, D. [@realDonaldTrump]. (2020, October 6c). *New FDA Rules make it more difficult for them to speed up vaccines for approval before Election Day. Just another political hit job! @SteveFDA* [Tweet]. Trump archiver. https://bit.ly/3syCKue

Trump, D. [@realDonaldTrump]. (2020, October 7). *My highly regarded Executive Order protected 525,000 American jobs during the height of the Chinese Plague. Democrats want to have Open Borders!* [Tweet]. Trump archiver. https://bit.ly/3syCKue

Trump, D. [@realDonaldTrump]. (2020, October 12). *The World Health Organization just admitted that I was right. Lockdowns are killing countries all over the world. The cure cannot be worse than the problem itself. Open up your states, Democrat governors. Open up New York. A long battle, but they finally did the right thing!* [Tweet]. Trump archiver. https://bit.ly/3syCKue

Trump, D. [@realDonaldTrump]. (2020, October 13). *Totally Negative China Virus Reports. Hit it early and hard. Fake News is devastated. They are very bad (and sick!) people!* [Tweet]. Trump archiver. https://bit.ly/3syCKue

Trump, D. [@realDonaldTrump]. (2020, October 18). *Totally Negative China Virus Reports. Hit it early and hard. Fake News is devastated. They are very bad (and sick!) people!* [Tweet]. Trump archiver. https://bit.ly/3syCKue

Trump, D. [@realDonaldTrump]. (2020, October 21). *....Should take care of our people. It wasn't their fault that the Plague came in from China!* [Tweet]. Trump archiver. https://bit.ly/3syCKue

Trump, D. [@realDonaldTrump]. (2020, October 23). *Joe Biden's response to the H1N1 Swine Flu, far less lethal than Covid 19, was one of the weakest and worst in the history of fighting epidemics and pandemics. It was pathetic, those involved have said. Joe didn't have a clue!* [Tweet]. Trump archiver. https://bit.ly/3syCKue

Trump, D. [@realDonaldTrump]. (2020, October 26). *We have made tremendous progress with the China Virus, but the Fake News refuses to talk about it this close to the Election. COVID, COVID, COVID is being used by them, in total coordination, in order to change our great early election numbers.Should be an election law violation!* [Tweet]. Trump archiver. https://bit.ly/3syCKue

Trump, D. [@realDonaldTrump]. (2020, October 27a). *Death rate of people going into hospitals is MUCH LOWER now than it was. @MSNBC Wow, MSDNC has come a long way! The fact is that we have learned and done a lot about this Virus. Much different now than when it first arrived on our shores, and the World's, from China!* [Tweet]. Trump archiver. https://bit.ly/3syCKue

Trump, D. [@realDonaldTrump]. (2020, October 27b). *This election is a choice between a TRUMP RECOVERY or a BIDEN DEPRESSION. It's a choice between a TRUMP BOOM or a BIDEN LOCKDOWN. It's a choice between our plan to Kill the virus – or Biden's plan to kill the American Dream! https://t.co/DreEqXJMNu* [Tweet]. Trump archiver. https://bit.ly/3syCKue

Trump, D. [@realDonaldTrump]. (2020, October 28). *This election is a choice between a TRUMP RECOVERY or a BIDEN DEPRESSION. It's a choice between a TRUMP*

*BOOM or a BIDEN LOCKDOWN. It's a choice between our plan to Kill the virus – or Biden's plan to kill the American Dream! https://t.co/DreEqXJMNu* [Tweet]. Trump archiver. https://bit.ly/3syCKue

Trump, D. J. [@realDonaldTrump]. (2020, October 30). *This election is a choice between a Trump Super Boom or a Biden Depression, and it's between a safe vaccine or a devastating Biden lockdown! https://t.co/FkOHz0XUS2 https://t.co/IEPULUXAXe* [Tweet]. Trump archiver. https://bit.ly/3syCKue

Trump, D. [@realDonaldTrump]. (2020, November 1). *Biden wants to LOCKDOWN our Country, maybe for years. Crazy! There will be NO LOCKDOWNS. The great American Comeback is underway!!!* [Tweet]. Trump archiver. https://bit.ly/3syCKue

Trump, D. [@realDonaldTrump]. (2020, November 9). *As I have long said, @Pfizer and the others would only announce a Vaccine after the Election, because they didn't have the courage to do it before. Likewise, the @US_FDA should have announced it earlier, not for political purposes, but for saving lives!* [Tweet]. Trump archiver. https://bit.ly/3syCKue

Trump, D. [@realDonaldTrump]. (2020, November 10). *WATCH FOR MASSIVE BALLOT COUNTING ABUSE AND, JUST LIKE THE EARLY VACCINE, REMEMBER I TOLD YOU SO!* [Tweet]. Trump archiver. https://bit.ly/3syCKue

Trump, D. [@realDonaldTrump]. (2020, November 16). *Another Vaccine just announced. This time by Moderna, 95% effective. For those great "historians", please remember that these great discoveries, which will end the China Plague, all took place on my watch!* [Tweet]. Trump archiver. https://bit.ly/3syCKue

Trump, D. [@realDonaldTrump]. (2020, November 21). *Fake News always "forgets" to mention that far fewer people are dying when they get Covid. This is do to both our advanced therapeutics, and the gained knowledge of our great doctors, nurses and front line workers!* [Tweet]. Trump archiver. https://bit.ly/3syCKue

Trump, D. [@realDonaldTrump]. (2020, November 22). *Report: Maryland Gov. Larry Hogan, Anti-Trump Hero, Paid for Flawed Coronavirus Tests from South Korea https://t.co/PHV7euutVb via @BreitbartNews. This RINO will never make the grade. Hogan is just as bad as the flawed tests he paid big money for!* [Tweet]. Trump archiver. https://bit.ly/3syCKue

Trump, D. [@realDonaldTrump]. (2020, November 30). *Moderna now applying for Emergency Vaccine Approval.. @US_FDA MUST ACT QUICKLY!!! "Operation Warp Speed has been a great modern day miracle."* [Tweet]. Trump archiver. https://bit.ly/3syCKue

Trump, D. [@realDonaldTrump]. (2020, December 9). *Germany has consistently been used by my obnoxious critics as the country that we should follow on the way to handle the China Virus. So much for that argument. I love Germany - Vaccines on the way!!! https://t.co/hEeKIqDMQn* [Tweet]. Trump archiver. https://bit.ly/3syCKue

Trump, D. [@realDonaldTrump]. (2020, December 11a). *While my pushing the money drenched but heavily bureaucratic @US_FDA saved five years in the approval of NUMEROUS great new vaccines, it is still a big, old, slow turtle. Get the dam vaccines out NOW, Dr. Hahn @SteveFDA. Stop playing games and start saving lives!!!* [Tweet]. Trump archiver. https://bit.ly/3syCKue

Trump, D. [@realDonaldTrump]. (2020, December 11b). "*Donald Trump must get the credit for the vaccines. It is a miracle." @Varneyco* [Tweet]. Trump archiver. https://bit.ly/3syCKue

Trump, D. [@realDonaldTrump]. (2020, December 18). "*Europe and other parts of the World being hit hard by the China Virus - Germany, France, Spain and Italy, in particular. The vaccines are on their way!!!* [Tweet]. Trump archiver. https://bit.ly/3syCKu

Trump, D. [@realDonaldTrump]. (2020, December 19). *The entire WORLD is being badly hurt by the China Virus, but if you listen to the Fake News Lamestream Media, and*

*Big Tech, you would think that we are the only one. No, but we are the Country that developed vaccines, and years ahead of schedule! https://t.co/z1UoJ8lbTm* [Tweet]. Trump archiver. https://bit.ly/3syCKu

Trump, D. J. [@realDonaldTrump]. (2020, December 22). *Distribution of both vaccines is going very smoothly. Amazing how many people are being vaccinated, record numbers. Our Country, and indeed the World, will soon see the great miracle of what the Trump Administration has accomplished. They said it couldn't be done!!!* [Tweet]. Trump archiver. https://bit.ly/3syCKue

Trump, D. [@realDonaldTrump]. (2020, December 29). *$2000 for our great people, not $600! They have suffered enough from the China Virus!!!* [Tweet]. Trump archiver. https://bit.ly/3syCKu

Trump, D. [@realDonaldTrump]. (2021, January 3). *The number of cases and deaths of the China Virus is far exaggerated in the United States because of @CDCgov's ridiculous method of determination compared to other countries, many of whom report, purposely, very inaccurately and low. "When in doubt, call it Covid." Fake News!* [Tweet]. Trump archiver. https://bit.ly/3syCKu

Trump, D. [@realDonaldTrump]. (2020, March 11b). *The Media should view this as a time of unity and strength. We have a common enemy, actually, an enemy of the World, the CoronaVirus. We must beat it as quickly and safely as possible. There is nothing more important to me than the life & safety of the United States!* [Tweet]. Trump archiver. https://bit.ly/3syCKue

Trump, D. [@realDonaldTrump]. (2020, March 11c). *I am fully prepared to use the full power of the Federal Government to deal with our current challenge of the CoronaVirus!* [Tweet]. Trump archiver. https://bit.ly/3syCKue

Trump, D. [@realDonaldTrump]. (2020, March 12). *108 countries are dealing with the CoronaVirus problem, some of which we are helping!* [Tweet]. Trump archiver. https://bit.ly/3syCKue

Trump, D. [@realDonaldTrump]. (2020, March 13a). *To this point, and because we have had a very strong border policy, we have had 40 deaths related to CoronaVirus. If we had weak or open borders, that number would be many times higher!* [Tweet]. Trump archiver. https://bit.ly/3syCKue

Trump, D. [@realDonaldTrump]. (2020, March 13b). *For decades the @CDCgov looked at, and studied, its testing system, but did nothing about it. It would always be inadequate and slow for a large scale pandemic, but a pandemic would never happen, they hoped. President Obama made changes that only complicated things further* [Tweet]. Trump archiver. https://bit.ly/3syCKue

Trump, D. [@realDonaldTrump]. (2020, March 14a). *SOCIAL DISTANCING!* [Tweet]. Trump archiver. https://bit.ly/3syCKue

Trump, D. [@realDonaldTrump]. (2020, March 14b). *Just had a nice conversation with Prime Minister @JustinTrudeau of Canada. Great to hear that his wonderful wife Sophie is doing very well. The United States and Canada will continue to coordinate closely together on COVID-19* [Tweet]. Trump archiver. https://bit.ly/3syCKue

Trump, D. [@realDonaldTrump]. (2020, March 15a). *The USA was never set up for this, just look at the catastrophe of the H1N1 Swine Flu (Biden in charge, 17,000 people lost, very late response time), but it soon will be. Great decision to close our China, and other, borders early. Saved many lives!* [Tweet]. Trump archiver. https://bit.ly/3syCKue

Trump, D. [@realDonaldTrump]. (2020, March 15b). *I am proud to announce that the United States will donate ventilators to our friends in India. We stand with India and @narendramodi during this pandemic. We're also cooperating on vaccine development. Together we will beat the invisible enemy!* [Tweet]. Trump archiver. https://bit.ly/3syCKue

Trump, D. [@realDonaldTrump]. (2020, March 16). *The United States will be powerfully supporting those industries, like Airlines and others, that are particularly affected by the*

*Chinese Virus. We will be stronger than ever before!* [Tweet]. Trump archiver. https://bit.ly/3syCKue

Trump, D. [@realDonaldTrump]. (2020, March 18b). *I only signed the Defense Production Act to combat the Chinese Virus should we need to invoke it in a worst case scenario in the future. Hopefully there will be no need, but we are all in this TOGETHER!* [Tweet]. Trump archiver. https://bit.ly/3syCKue

Trump, D. [@realDonaldTrump]. (2020, March 18a). *For the people that are now out of work because of the important and necessary containment policies, for instance the shutting down of hotels, bars and restaurants, money will soon be coming to you. The onslaught of the Chinese Virus is not your fault! Will be stronger than ever!* [Tweet]. Trump archiver. https://bit.ly/3syCKue

Trump, D. [@realDonaldTrump]. (2020, March 19*). SOCIAL DISTANCING! https://t.co/H2jR59wArx* [Tweet]. Trump archiver. https://bit.ly/3syCKue

Trump, D. [@realDonaldTrump]. (2020, March 21). *HYDROXYCHLOROQUINE & AZITHROMYCIN, taken together, have a real chance to be one of the biggest game changers in the history of medicine. The FDA has moved mountains - Thank You! Hopefully they will BOTH (H works better with A, International Journal of Antimicrobial Agents)* [Tweet]. Trump archiver. https://bit.ly/3syCKue

Trump, D. [@realDonaldTrump]. (2020, March 23b). *It is very important that we totally protect our Asian American community in the United States, and all around the world. They are amazing people, and the spreading of the Virus is not their fault in any way, shape, or form. They are working closely with us to get rid of it. WE WILL PREVAIL TOGETHER!* [Tweet]. Trump archiver. https://bit.ly/3syCKue

Trump, D. [@realDonaldTrump]. (2020, March 24). *Our people want to return to work. They will practice Social Distancing and all else, and Seniors will be watched over protectively & lovingly. We can do two things together. THE CURE CANNOT BE*

*WORSE (by far) THAN THE PROBLEM! Congress MUST ACT NOW. We will come back strong!* [Tweet]. Trump archiver. https://bit.ly/3syCKue

Trump, D. [@realDonaldTrump]. (2020, March 27). *We are marshalling the full power of government and society to achieve victory over the virus. Together, we will endure, we will prevail, and we will WIN! #CARESAct https://t.co/zb2PJTldGQ* [Tweet]. Trump archiver. https://bit.ly/3syCKue

Trump, D. [@realDonaldTrump]. (2020, March 30). *We are marshalling the full power of government and society to achieve victory over the virus. Together, we will endure, we will prevail, and we will WIN! #CARESAct https://t.co/zb2PJTldGQ* [Tweet]. Trump archiver. https://bit.ly/3syCKue

Trump, D. [@realDonaldTrump]. (2020, April 7). *The W.H.O. really blew it. For some reason, funded largely by the United States, yet very China centric. We will be giving that a good look. Fortunately I rejected their advice on keeping our borders open to China early on. Why did they give us such a faulty recommendation?* [Tweet]. Trump archiver. https://bit.ly/3syCKue

Trump, D. [@realDonaldTrump]. (2020, April 9). *.@OANN A key CoronaVirus Model is now predicting far fewer deaths than the number shown in earlier models. That's because the American people are doing a great job. Social Distancing etc. Keep going!* [Tweet]. Trump archiver. https://bit.ly/3syCKue

Trump, D. [@realDonaldTrump]. (2020, April 11). *So now the Fake News @nytimes is tracing the CoronaVirus origins back to Europe, NOT China. This is a first! I wonder what the Failing New York Times got for this one? Are there any NAMED sources? They were recently thrown out of China like dogs, and obviously want back in. Sad!* [Tweet]. Trump archiver. https://bit.ly/3syCKue

Trump, D. [@realDonaldTrump]. (2020, April 17). *Why did the W.H.O. Ignore an email from Taiwanese health officials in late December alerting them to the possibility that CoronaVirus could be transmitted between humans? Why did the W.H.O. make several claims about the CoronaVirus that ere either inaccurate or misleading* [Tweet]. Trump archiver. https://bit.ly/3syCKue

Trump, D. [@realDonaldTrump]. (2020, April 17). *Why did the W.H.O. Ignore an email from Taiwanese health officials in late December alerting them to the possibility that CoronaVirus could be transmitted between humans? Why did the W.H.O. make several claims about the CoronaVirus that ere either inaccurate or misleading* [Tweet]. Trump archiver. https://bit.ly/3syCKue

Trump, D. [@realDonaldTrump]. (2020, April 18). *..them happy, or even a little bit satisfied. They were RUDE and NASTY. This is their political playbook, and they will use it right up to the election on November 3rd. They will not change because they feel that this is the only way they can win. America will not be fooled!!!* [Tweet]. Trump archiver. https://bit.ly/3syCKue

Trump, D. [@realDonaldTrump]. (2020, April 22). *CDC Director was totally misquoted by Fake News @CNN on Covid 19. He will be putting out a statement* [Tweet]. Trump archiver. https://bit.ly/3syCKue

Trump, D. [@realDonaldTrump]. (2020, April 24). *Great conversation with President Lenin Moreno of the Republic of Ecuador. We will be sending them desperately needed Ventilators, of which we have recently manufactured many, and helping them in other ways. They are fighting hard against CoronaVirus!* [Tweet]. Trump archiver. https://bit.ly/3syCKue

Trump, D. [@realDonaldTrump]. (2020, April 25). *The Do Nothing Democrats are spending much of their money on Fake Ads. I never said that the CoronaVirus is a "Hoax", I said that the Democrats, and the way they lied about it, are a Hoax. Also, it did start with "one person from China", and then grew, & will be a "Miracle" end!* [Tweet]. Trump archiver. https://bit.ly/3syCKue

Trump, D. [@realDonaldTrump]. (2020, April 29). *The only reason the U.S. has reported one million cases of CoronaVirus is that our Testing is sooo much better than any other country in the World. Other countries are way behind us in Testing, and therefore show far fewer cases!* [Tweet]. Trump archiver. https://bit.ly/3syCKue

Trump, D. [@realDonaldTrump]. (2020, April 30). *Despite reports to the contrary, Sweden is paying heavily for its decision not to lockdown. As of today, 2462 people have died there, a much higher number than the neighboring countries of Norway (207), Finland (206) or Denmark (443). The United States made the correct decision!* [Tweet]. Trump archiver. https://bit.ly/3syCKue

Trump, D. [@realDonaldTrump]. (2020, May 2). *The Democrats are just, as always, looking for trouble. They do nothing constructive, even in times of crisis. They don't want to blame their cash cow, China, for the plague. China is blaming Europe. Dr. Fauci will be testifying before the Senate very soon! #DONOTHINGDEMOCRATS https://t.co/fgHuYeiOQY* [Tweet]. Trump archiver. https://bit.ly/3syCKue

Trump, D. [@realDonaldTrump]. (2020, May 2). *The Democrats are just, as always, looking for trouble. They do nothing constructive, even in times of crisis. They don't want to blame their cash cow, China, for the plague. China is blaming Europe. Dr. Fauci will be testifying before the Senate very soon! #DONOTHINGDEMOCRATS https://t.co/fgHuYeiOQY* [Tweet]. Trump archiver. https://bit.ly/3syCKue

Trump, D. [@realDonaldTrump]. (2020, May 4). *Mexico is sadly experiencing very big CoronaVirus problems, and now California, get this, doesn't want people coming over the Southern Border. A Classic! They are sooo lucky that I am their President. Border is very tight and the Wall is rapidly being built!* [Tweet]. Trump archiver. https://bit.ly/3syCKue

Trump, D. [@realDonaldTrump]. (2020, May 6). *....to it, as appropriate. The Task Force will also be very focused on Vaccines & Therapeutics. Thank you!* [Tweet]. Trump archiver. https://bit.ly/3syCKue

Trump, D. [@realDonaldTrump]. (2020, May 10a). *We are getting great marks for the handling of the CoronaVirus pandemic, especially the very early BAN of people from*

*China, the infectious source, entering the USA. Compare that to the Obama/Sleepy Joe disaster known as H1N1 Swine Flu. Poor marks, bad polls - didn't have a clue!* [Tweet]. Trump archiver. https://bit.ly/3syCKue

Trump, D. [@realDonaldTrump]. (2020, May 10b). *@CBS and their show, @60Minutes, are doing everything within their power, which is far less today than it was in the past, to defend China and the horrible Virus pandemic that was inflicted on the USA and the rest of the World. I guess they want to do business in China!* [Tweet]. Trump archiver. https://bit.ly/3syCKue

Trump, D. [@realDonaldTrump]. (2020, May 15). *I am proud to announce that the United States will donate ventilators to our friends in India. We stand with India and @narendramodi during this pandemic. We're also cooperating on vaccine development. Together we will beat the invisible enemy!* [Tweet]. Trump archiver. https://bit.ly/3syCKue

Trump, D. [@realDonaldTrump]. (2020, May 16). *.....are therefore given massive advantages over The United States, and everyone else? Prior to the Plague floating in from China, our Economy was blowing everybody away, the best of any country, EVER. We will be there again, and soon!* [Tweet]. Trump archiver. https://bit.ly/3syCKue

Trump, D. [@realDonaldTrump]. (2020, May 20).....*It all comes from the top. They could have easily stopped the plague, but they didn't!* [Tweet]. Trump archiver. https://bit.ly/3syCKue

Trump, D. [@realDonaldTrump]. (2020, May 26). *....One person lost to this invisible virus is too much, it should have been stopped at its source, China, but I acted very quickly, and made the right decisions. Many of the current political complainers thought, at the time, that I was moving far to fast, like Crazy Nancy!* [Tweet]. Trump archiver. https://bit.ly/3syCKue

Trump, D. [@realDonaldTrump]. (2020, May 27). *The Radical Left Lamestream Media, together with their partner, the Do Nothing Democrats, are trying to spread a new narrative that President Trump was slow in reacting to Covid 19. Wrong, I was very fast, even doing the Ban on China long before anybody thought necessary!* [Tweet]. Trump archiver. https://bit.ly/3syCKue

Trump, D. [@realDonaldTrump]. (2020, May 28). *All over the World the CoronaVirus, a very bad "gift" from China, marches on. Not good!* [Tweet]. Trump archiver. https://bit.ly/3syCKue

Trump, D. [@realDonaldTrump]. (2020, May 29). *The Radical Left Lamestream Media, together with their partner, the Do Nothing Democrats, are trying to spread a new narrative that President Trump was slow in reacting to Covid 19. Wrong, I was very fast, even doing the Ban on China long before anybody thought necessary!* [Tweet]. Trump archiver. https://bit.ly/3syCKue

Trump, D. [@realDonaldTrump]. (2020, June 2). *Vaccines are coming along really well. Likewise therapeutics. Moving faster than anticipated. Good news ahead (in many ways)!* [Tweet]. Trump archiver. https://bit.ly/3syCKue

Trump, D. [@realDonaldTrump]. (2020, June 19). *Tony Fauci has nothing to do with NFL Football. They are planning a very safe and controlled opening. However, if they don't stand for our National Anthem and our Great American Flag, I won't be watching!!!* [Tweet]. Trump archiver. https://bit.ly/3syCKue

Trump, D. [@realDonaldTrump]. (2020, June 22a). *Because of MAIL-IN BALLOTS, 2020 will be the most RIGGED Election in our nations history - unless this stupidity is ended. We voted during World War One & World War Two with no problem, but now they are using Covid in order to cheat by using Mail-Ins!* [Tweet]. Trump archiver. https://bit.ly/3syCKue

Trump, D. [@realDonaldTrump]. (2020, June 22b). *"His (President Trump's) policies set a foundation that allowed us to survive the pandemic." @HeyTammyBruce @SteveHiltonx @FoxNews True, we built something so strong that we are now setting economic growth records again - Jobs & Growth!!! [Tweet].* Trump archiver. https://bit.ly/3syCKue

Trump, D. [@realDonaldTrump]. (2020, June 25). *Coronavirus deaths are way down. Mortality rate is one of the lowest in the World. Our Economy is roaring back and will NOT be shut down. "Embers" or flare ups will be put out, as necessary!* [Tweet]. Trump archiver. https://bit.ly/3syCKue

Trump, D. [@realDonaldTrump]. (2020, June 27). *Corrupt Joe Biden said yesterday that we have over "120 million" people dead of Coronavirus!* [Tweet]. Trump archiver. https://bit.ly/3syCKue

Trump, D. [@realDonaldTrump]. (2020, June 30). *As I watch the Pandemic spread its ugly face all across the world, including the tremendous damage it has done to the USA, I become more and more angry at China. People can see it, and I can feel it!* [Tweet]. Trump archiver. https://bit.ly/3syCKue

Trump, D. [@realDonaldTrump]. (2020, July 6a). *Why does the Lamestream Fake News Media REFUSE to say that China Virus deaths are down 39%, and that we now have the lowest Fatality (Mortality) Rate in the World. They just can't stand that we are doing so well for our Country!* [Tweet]. Trump archiver. https://bit.ly/3syCKue

Trump, D. [@realDonaldTrump]. (2020, July 6b). *The highly respected Henry Ford Health System just reported, based on a large sampling, that HYDROXYCHLOROQUINE cut the death rate in certain sick patients very significantly. The Dems disparaged it for political reasons (me!). Disgraceful. Act now @US_FDA @TuckerCarlson @FoxNews* [Tweet]. Trump archiver. https://bit.ly/3syCKue

Trump, D. [@realDonaldTrump]. (2020, July 7). *"COVID-19 (China Virus) Death Rate PLUNGES From Peak In U.S." A Tenfold Decrease In Mortality. The Washington Times @WashTimes Valerie Richardson. We have the lowest Mortality Rate in the World. The Fake News should be reporting these most important of facts, but they don't!* [Tweet]. Trump archiver. https://bit.ly/3syCKue

Trump, D. [@realDonaldTrump]. (2020, March 5d). *"I want to commend the President for how he has handled the CoronaVirus situation, especially his early decision to shut down access into our Country from China, despite strong opposition to that decision." @SenTomCotton Thank you Tom!* [Tweet]. Trump archiver. https://bit.ly/3syCKue

Trump, D. [@realDonaldTrump]. (2020, March 8). *We have a perfectly coordinated and fine tuned plan at the White House for our attack on CoronaVirus. We moved VERY early to close borders to certain areas, which was a Godsend. V.P. is doing a great job. The Fake News Media is doing everything possible to make us look bad. Sad!* [Tweet]. Trump archiver. https://bit.ly/3syCKue

Trump, D. [@realDonaldTrump]. (2020, March 9a). *The Fake News Media and their partner, the Democrat Party, is doing everything within its semi-considerable power (it used to be greater!) to inflame the CoronaVirus situation, far beyond what the facts would warrant. Surgeon General, "The risk is low to the average American."* [Tweet]. Trump archiver. https://bit.ly/3syCKue

Trump, D. [@realDonaldTrump]. (2020, March 9b). *So last year 37,000 Americans died from the common Flu. It averages between 27,000 and 70,000 per year. Nothing is shut down, life & the economy go on. At this moment there are 546 confirmed cases of CoronaVirus, with 22 deaths. Think about that!* [Tweet]. Trump archiver. https://bit.ly/3syCKue

Trump, D. [@realDonaldTrump]. (2020, March 11a). *America is the Greatest Country in the world. We have the best scientists, doctors, nurses and health care professionals. They are amazing people who do phenomenal things every day* [Tweet]. Trump archiver. https://bit.ly/3syCKue

Trump, D. [ABC News]. (2017, January 20*). Trump Inauguration Speech (FULL)* [Video]. https://www.youtube.com/watch?v=sRBsJNdK1t0

Trump, D. & Schwartz, T. (1987). *Trump: The Art of the Deal*. Random House.

Trump, D. J. [@realDonaldTrump]. (2020, March 21). *"HYDROXYCHLOROQUINE & AZITHROMYCIN, taken together, have a real chance to be one of the biggest game changers in the history of medicine. The FDA has moved mountains—Thank You!"* [Tweet]. Trump archiver. https://bit.ly/3syCKue

Trump, D. J. [@realDonaldTrump]. (2020, October). *Covid, Covid, Covid is the unified chant of the Fake News Lamestream Media. They will talk about nothing else until November 4th., when the Election will be (hopefully!) over. Then the talk will be how low the death rate is, plenty of hospital rooms, & many tests of young people* [Tweet]. Trump archiver. https://bit.ly/3syCKue

Trump, D. J. [@realDonaldTrump]. (2020, September 29). *If we listened to Joe Biden on coronavirus, millions of people would have died!* [Tweet]. Trump archiver. https://bit.ly/3syCKue

Tuchman, G. (1978). *Making news: A study in the construction of reality* . The Free Press.

Tversky, A., & Kahneman, D. (1981). The framing of decisions and the psychology of choice. *science*, 211(4481), 453-458.

TweetBinder (2020, n.d.). *Donald Trump and Twitter – 2009 / 2021 analysis*. Tweetbinder. https://www.tweetbinder.com/blog/trump-twitter/

Twitter (2021, January 8). *Permanent suspension of @realDonaldTrump*. Twitter https://blog.twitter.com/en_us/topics/company/2020/suspension.html

Twitter (n.d b). *How to create a thread on Twitter and how to view*. Twitter. https://help.twitter.com/en/using-twitter/create-a-thread#:~:text=Sometimes%20we%20need%20more%20than,by%20connecting%20multiple%20Tweets%20together.

Twitter (n.d.). *About your Twitter timeline*. Twitter. https://help.twitter.com/en/using-twitter/twitter-timeline#:~:text=Your%20Home%20timeline%20displays%20a,chosen%20to%20follow

%20on%20Twitter.&text=You%20can%20reply%2C%20Retweet%2C%20or,for%20iOS%20and%20Android%20only

U.S. Food and Drug Administration Coronavirus [FDA] (2020, April 24). *(COVID-19) Update: FDA Reiterates Importance of Close Patient Supervision for 'Off-Label' Use of Antimalarial Drugs to Mitigate Known Risks, Including Heart Rhythm Problems*. FDA. https://www.fda.gov/news-events/press-announcements/coronavirus-covid-19-update-fda-reiterates-importance-close-patient-supervision-label-use

USA Today (2020, n.d). *Read the full transcript from the first presidential debate between Joe Biden and Donald Trump*. USA Today News. https://eu.usatoday.com/story/news/politics/elections/2020/09/30/presidential-debate-read-full-transcript-first-debate/3587462001/

Van Bavel, J. J., Baicker, K., Boggio, P. S., Capraro, V., Cichocka, A., Cikara, M., ... & Willer, R. (2020). Using social and behavioural science to support COVID-19 pandemic response. *Nature human behaviour*, 4(5), 460-471.

Van Dick, R., Hirst, G., Grojean, M. W., & Wieseke, J. (2007). Relationships between leader and follower organizational identification and implications for follower attitudes and behaviour. *Journal of Occupational and Organizational Psychology*, 80(1), 133-150.

Van Dijk, T. A. (2006). Ideology and discourse analysis. *Journal of political ideologies*, 11(2), 115-140.

Van Gorp, B. (2010). *Strategies to take subjectivity out of framing analysis. Doing news framing analysis: Empirical and theoretical perspectives*, 84-109.

Van Hulst, M., & Yanow, D. (2016). From policy "frames" to "framing" theorizing a more dynamic, political approach. *The American review of public administration*, 46(1), 92-112.

Vargo, D., Zhu, L., Benwell, B., & Yan, Z. (2021). Digital technology use during COVID-19 pandemic: A rapid review. *Human Behavior and Emerging Technologies*, 3(1), 13-24.

Villa, S., Jaramillo, E., Mangioni, D., Bandera, A., Gori, A., & Raviglione, M. C. (2020). Stigma at the time of the COVID-19 pandemic. Clinical Microbiology and Infection, 26(11), 1450-1452.

Vliegenthart, R., & Van Zoonen, L. (2011). Power to the frame: Bringing sociology back to frame analysis. European journal of communication, 26(2), 101-115.

Wahyuningsih, S. (2018). A discourse analysis: Personal pronouns in Donald Trump's inauguration speech. In English Language and Literature International Conference (ELLiC) Proceedings (Vol. 2, pp. 346-350).

Wallis, P., & Nerlich, B. (2005). Disease metaphors in new epidemics: the UK media framing of the 2003 SARS epidemic. Social science & medicine, 60(11), 2629-2639.

Walsh, J. (18, October 17). 11 insults Trump has hurled at women. Business Insider. https://www.businessinsider.com/trumps-worst-insults-toward-women-2018-10?r=DE&IR=T

Wan (2020, March 11). *WHO declares a pandemic of coronavirus disease covid-19*. Washington Post. https://www.washingtonpost.com/health/2020/03/11/who-declares-pandemic-coronavirus-disease-covid-19/

Warren, E., Blumenthal, R. & Edward, J., M. (2020). *Letter to PRAC re politicization of COVID response*. ED Markey. https://www.markey.senate.gov/news/press-releases/warren-blumenthal-and-markey-urge-cares-act-inspectors-general-to-investigate-political-interference-in-trump-administrations-covid-19-response

Wasike, B. S. (2013). Framing News in 140 Characters: How Social Media Editors Frame the News and Interact with Audiences via Twitter. *Global Media Journal: Canadian Edition*, 6(1), 5-23.

Weaver, D. H. (2007). Thoughts on agenda setting, framing, and priming. *Journal of communication*, 57(1), 142-147.

Weber, R. P. (1990). *Basic content analysis* (No. 49). Sage.

Weiss, M. (1997). Signifying the pandemics: metaphors of AIDS, cancer, and heart disease. *Medical Anthropology Quarterly*, 11(4), 456–476.

Wells, C., Shah, D. V., Pevehouse, J. C., Yang, J., Pelled, A., Boehm, F., ... & Schmidt, J. L. (2016). How Trump drove coverage to the nomination: Hybrid media campaigning. *Political Communication*, 33(4), 669-676.

Wells, C., Shah, D., Lukito, J., Pelled, A., Pevehouse, J. C., & Yang, J. (2020). Trump, Twitter, and news media responsiveness: A media systems approach. *New Media & Society*, 22(4), 659-682.

Wellsby, M., Siakaluk, P. D., Pexman, P. M., & Owen, W. J. (2010). Some insults are easier to detect: The embodied insult detection effect. *Frontiers in Psychology*, 1, 198.

Wicke, P., & Bolognesi, M. M. (2020). Framing COVID-19: How we conceptualize and discuss the pandemic on Twitter. arXiv preprint arXiv:2004.06986.

Wimmer, A. (1997). Explaining xenophobia and racism: A critical review of current research approaches. *Ethnic and racial studies*, 20(1), 17-41.

Winberg, O. (2017). Insult politics: Donald Trump, right-wing populism, and incendiary language. *European journal of American studies*, 12(12-2).

Wojcik, S., Hughes, A., & Remy, E. (2019). *About one-in-five adult Twitter users in the US follow Trump*. Pew Research Center. https://www.pewresearch.org/fact-tank/2019/07/15/about-one-in-five-adult-twitter-users-in-the-u-s-follow-trump/

Worboys, M. (2000). *Spreading germs: disease, theories, and medical practice in Britain, 1865–1900.* Cambridge University Press.

World Health Organization (2015, May 8). *WHO issues best practices for naming new human infectious diseases. World health* organization. World Health Organization. https://www.who.int/news/item/08-05-2015-who-issues-best-practices-for-naming-new-human-infectious-diseases.

World Health Organization. (2020a). *Managing the COVID-19 infodemic: Promoting healthy behaviours and mitigating the harm from misinformation and disinformation.* World Health Organization. https://www.who.int/news/item/23-09-2020-managing-the-covid-19-infodemic-promoting-healthy-behaviours-and-mitigating-the-harm-from-misinformation-and-disinformation

World Health Organization. (2020b). *Social Stigma associated with COVID-19.* World Health Organization. https://www.who.int/docs/default-source/coronaviruse/covid19-stigma-guide.pdf

Wong, B. (2020, October 8). *People Who Lost Loved Ones To Coronavirus React To Trump's Tweet.* HuffPost. https://www.huffpost.com/entry/people-lost-loved-ones-coronavirus-trump-tweet_l_5f7dfa01c5b62e45eed529ba

Yakushko, O. (2009). Xenophobia: Understanding the roots and consequences of negative attitudes toward immigrants. *The Counseling Psychologist*, 37(1), 36-66.

Yamey, G., & Gonsalves, G. (2020). *Donald Trump: a political determinant of covid-19.* The BMJ. https://www.bmj.com/content/bmj/369/bmj.m1643.full.pdf

Yaqub, U. (2020). Tweeting During the Covid-19 Pandemic: Sentiment Analysis of Twitter Messages by President Trump. *Digital Government: Research and Practice*, 2(1), 1-7.

Yourish, K. & Buchanan, L. (2020, November 24). *Since Election Day, a Lot of Tweeting and Not Much Else for Trump.* New York Times. https://www.nytimes.com/interactive/2020/11/24/us/politics/trump-twitter-tweets-election-results.html

Yu, J., Lu, Y., & Muñoz-Justicia, J. (2020). Analyzing Spanish News Frames on Twitter during COVID-19—A Network Study of El País and El Mundo. International journal of environmental research and public health, 17(15), 5414.

Zaller, J. & Chiu, D. (1996). Government's little helper: US press coverage of foreign policy crises, 1945-1991. *Political Communication*, 13(4), 385-407.

Zaller, J. R. (1992). *The nature and origins of mass opinion*. Cambridge university press.

Zhang, Y. (2019, May*). Language in our time: an empirical analysis of hashtags. In The World Wide Web Conference* (pp. 2378-2389).

Zhang, Y., Wells, C., Wang, S., & Rohe, K. (2018). Attention and amplification in the hybrid media system: The composition and activity of Donald Trump's Twitter following during the 2016 presidential election. *New Media & Society*, 20(9), 3161-3182.

# 9 Appendix

**Timeline of COVID-19 pandemic in the US**

First time period (24 January - 10 March 2020)
Epidemic

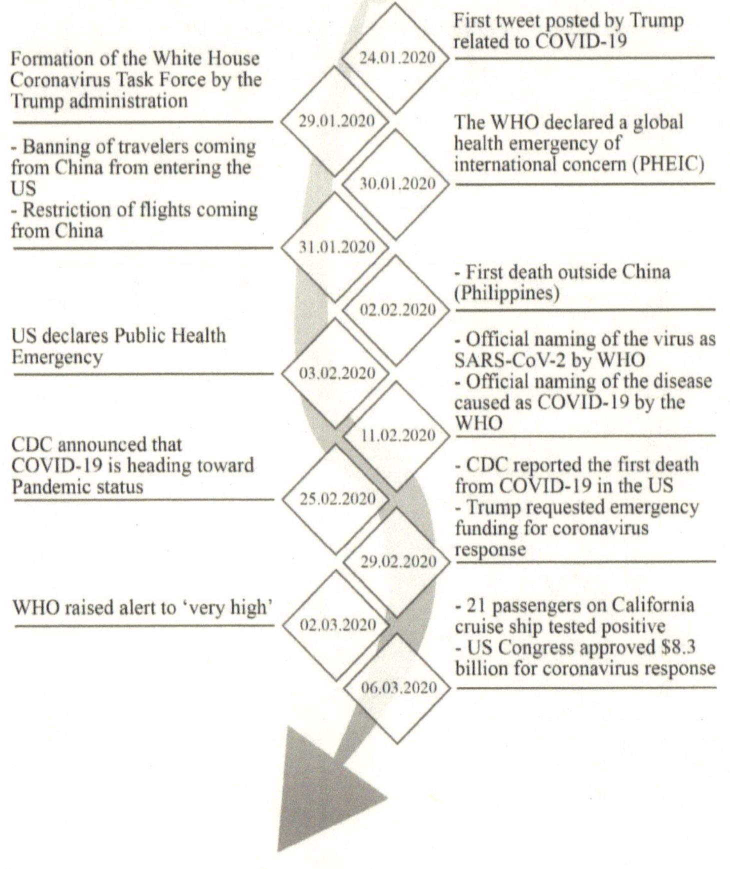

**Timeline of COVID-19 pandemic in the US**

Second time period ( 11 March - 28 September)
Pandemic (1/3)

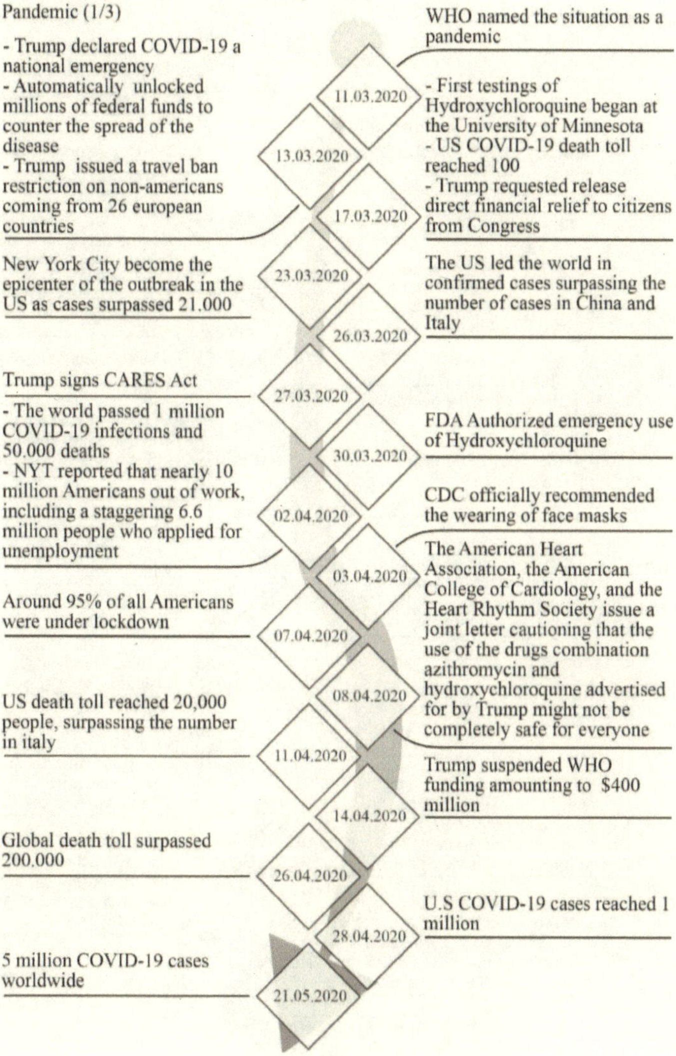

**Timeline of COVID-19 pandemic in the US**

Second time period ( 11 March - 28 September)
Pandemic (2/3)

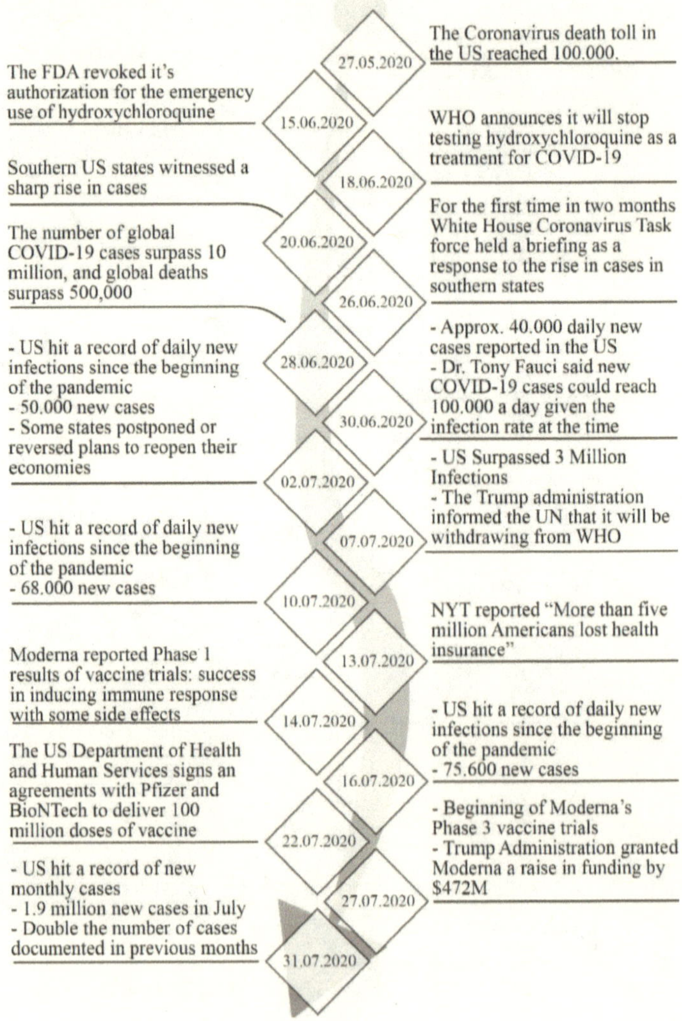

27.05.2020 — The Coronavirus death toll in the US reached 100.000.

15.06.2020 — The FDA revoked it's authorization for the emergency use of hydroxychloroquine

18.06.2020 — WHO announces it will stop testing hydroxychloroquine as a treatment for COVID-19

20.06.2020 — Southern US states witnessed a sharp rise in cases

26.06.2020 — For the first time in two months White House Coronavirus Task force held a briefing as a response to the rise in cases in southern states

28.06.2020 — The number of global COVID-19 cases surpass 10 million, and global deaths surpass 500,000

30.06.2020 — - Approx. 40.000 daily new cases reported in the US
- Dr. Tony Fauci said new COVID-19 cases could reach 100.000 a day given the infection rate at the time

02.07.2020 — - US hit a record of daily new infections since the beginning of the pandemic
- 50.000 new cases
- Some states postponed or reversed plans to reopen their economies

07.07.2020 — - US Surpassed 3 Million Infections
- The Trump administration informed the UN that it will be withdrawing from WHO

10.07.2020 — - US hit a record of daily new infections since the beginning of the pandemic
- 68.000 new cases

13.07.2020 — NYT reported "More than five million Americans lost health insurance"

14.07.2020 — Moderna reported Phase 1 results of vaccine trials: success in inducing immune response with some side effects

16.07.2020 — - US hit a record of daily new infections since the beginning of the pandemic
- 75.600 new cases

22.07.2020 — The US Department of Health and Human Services signs an agreements with Pfizer and BioNTech to deliver 100 million doses of vaccine

27.07.2020 — - Beginning of Moderna's Phase 3 vaccine trials
- Trump Administration granted Moderna a raise in funding by $472M

31.07.2020 — - US hit a record of new monthly cases
- 1.9 million new cases in July
- Double the number of cases documented in previous months

**Timeline of COVID-19 pandemic in the US**

Second time period ( 11 March - 28 September)
Pandemic (3/3)

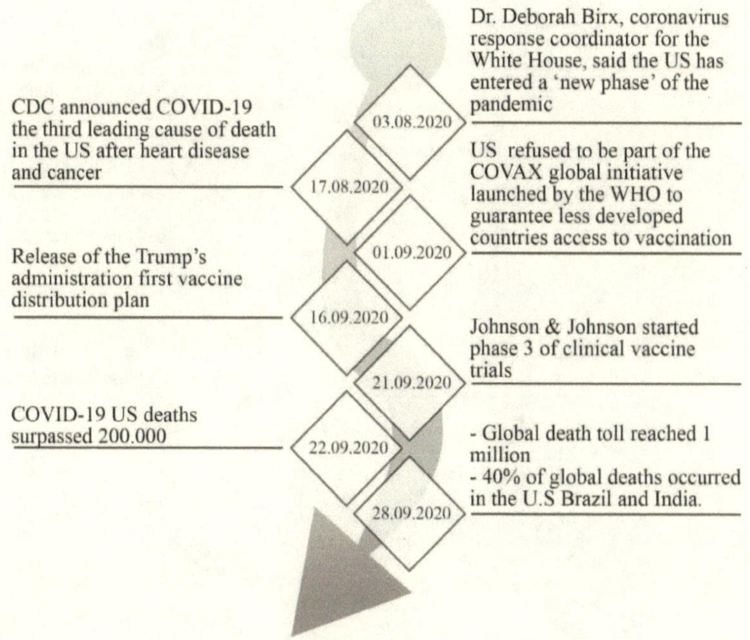

**Timeline of COVID-19 pandemic in the US**

Third time period (29 September - 3 November)
Pre-elections

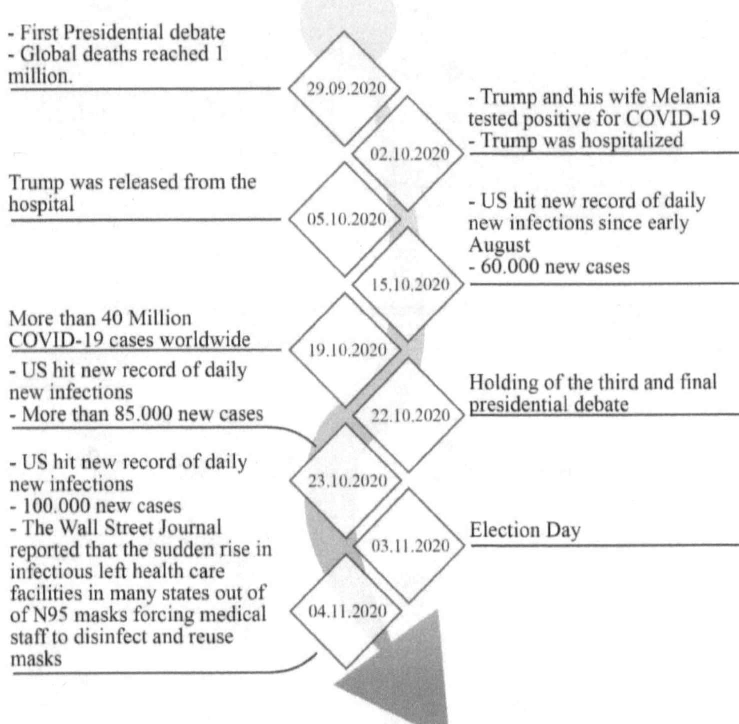

**Timeline of COVID-19 pandemic in the US**

Fourth time period ( 5 November - January 8)
Post elections

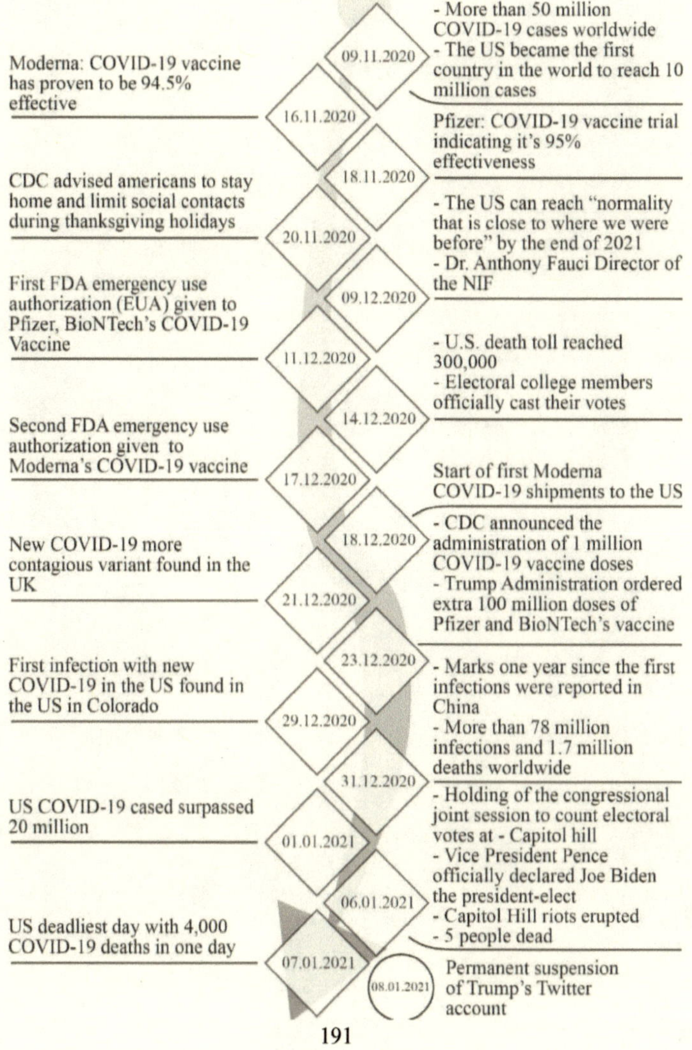

www.ingramcontent.com/pod-product-compliance
Lightning Source LLC
LaVergne TN
LVHW091315150826
845673LV00006B/1661

* 9 7 8 3 3 8 4 2 6 0 9 6 3 *